MW00718972

Mathematics:
With Allied Health Applications

Richard N. Aufmann
Palomar College

Joanne S. Lockwood
Nashua Community College

With Additional Contributions by
Catherine W. Johnson
Alamance Community College

Prepared by

Christine S. Verity

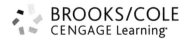
BROOKS/COLE
CENGAGE Learning

Australia • Brazil • Japan • Korea • Mexico • Singapore • Spain • United Kingdom • United States

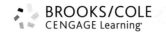

For product information and technology assistance, contact us at **Cengage Learning Customer & Sales Support, 1-800-354-9706**

For permission to use material from this text or product, submit all requests online at **www.cengage.com/permissions** Further permissions questions can be emailed to **permissionrequest@cengage.com**

ISBN-13: 978-1-133-11234-1
ISBN-10: 1-133-11234-X

Brooks/Cole
20 Davis Drive
Belmont, CA 94002-3098
USA

Cengage Learning is a leading provider of customized learning solutions with office locations around the globe, including Singapore, the United Kingdom, Australia, Mexico, Brazil, and Japan. Locate your local office at: **www.cengage.com/global**

Cengage Learning products are represented in Canada by Nelson Education, Ltd.

To learn more about Brooks/Cole, visit **www.cengage.com/brookscole**

Purchase any of our products at your local college store or at our preferred online store **www.cengagebrain.com**

Printed in the United States of America
1 2 3 4 5 6 7 15 14 13 12 11

Contents

Name   Score

Graph the number on the number line.

1. 2

2. 6

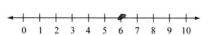

3. 7

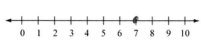

4. 1

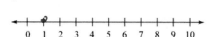

1. _____

2. _____

3. _____

4. _____

Place the correct symbol, < or >, between the two numbers.

5. 54 $>$ 47

6. 29 $>$ 11

7. 96 $<$ 97

8. 9 $<$ 13

9. 391 $>$ 250

10. 1010 $<$ 1110

11. 1 $<$ 64

12. 105 $>$ 0

13. 666 $<$ 777

14. 32,000 $>$ 3200

15. 5910 $>$ 5901

16. 63,528 $<$ 64,249

5. _____

6. _____

7. _____

8. _____

9. _____

10. _____

11. _____

12. _____

13. _____

14. _____

15. _____

16. _____

1

Name _____   Score _____

Write the number in words.

1. 862   2. 308   3. 654   1. _____

                                                                        2. _____

                                                                        3. _____

4. 5125   5. 9040   6. 36,844   4. _____

                                                                        5. _____

                                                                        6. _____

7. 380,751   8. 800,001   9. 7,640,723   7. _____

                                                                        8. _____

                                                                        9. _____

Write the number in standard form.

10. Thirty-three   11. Two hundred sixty-four   10. __33__

                                                                        11. __264__

12. Nine thousand five hundred 13. Fifty-six thousand three hundred 12. __9,527__
     twenty-seven   twenty
                                                                        13. _____

14. Four hundred sixty thousand 15. Four million twelve thousand   14. _____
     three hundred three   nine hundred eighty-six
                                                                        15. _____

16. One million five   17. Eight million one thousand fifty   16. _____

                                                                        17. _____

Name _____ Score _____

Write the number in expanded form.

1. 256

2. 4703

3. 9233

4. 23,040

5. 50,916

6. 75,049

7. 99,002

8. 234,782

9. 500,400

10. 787,000

11. 806,008

12. 920,010

13. 4,271,020

14. 6,000,213

1. _____

2. _____

3. _____

4. _____

5. _____

6. _____

7. _____

8. _____

9. _____

10. _____

11. _____

12. _____

13. _____

14. _____

Name   Score

Round the number to the given place value.

1.   747   Tens   2.   711   Tens   1. _____

                                                           2. _____

3.   361   Hundreds   4.   589   Hundreds   3. _____

                                                            4. _____

5.   1050   Hundreds   6.   7149   Hundreds   5. _____

                                                            6. _____

7.   4461   Thousands   8.   9620   Thousands   7. _____

                                                            8. _____

9.   74,510   Thousands   10.   69,372   Thousands   9. _____

                                                        10. _____

11.   250,650   Ten-thousands   12.   841,512   Ten-thousands   11. _____

                                                        12. _____

13.   3,467,000   Millions   14.   7,600,475   Millions   13. _____

                                                        14. _____

Name _____   Score _____

Add.

1.   391
     + 475

2.   568
     + 284

3.   821
     + 1774

4.   8515
      5307
     + 4518

5.   7810
      9537
     + 3284

6.   9478
      3925
     + 6227

7.   1982
      7650
      4319
     + 3766

8.   6452
      3339
      2751
     + 8892

9.   9655
      2356
      8878
     + 1664

10. 19,600
     45,328
     69,871
     24,443
    + 72,550

11. 36,450
     88,718
     30,957
     56,329
    + 94,005

12. 77,653
     82,280
     11,999
     70,554
    + 25,393

13. 567 + 23 + 849

14. 723 + 96 + 452

15. 4689 + 574 + 28,976

16. 2762 + 749 + 69,858

17. 465 + 8907 + 5293 + 51

18. 118 + 6447 + 9549 + 26

19. 35 + 8701 + 65,247 + 765

20. 48 + 7449 + 26,835 + 98

21.   39,153
         877
       5,442
       2,986
      43,298
     +   660

22.   6,471
     8,889,988
       19,927
           34
       45,638
     +   345

1. _____
2. _____
3. _____
4. _____
5. _____
6. _____
7. _____
8. _____
9. _____
10. _____
11. _____
12. _____
13. _____
14. _____
15. _____
16. _____
17. _____
18. _____
19. _____
20. _____
21. _____
22. _____

Name _____   Score _____

Solve.

1. You paid $67 for a coat and $14 for a hat.   2. A homemaker has a monthly budget of   1. _____
    Find the total cost of the coat and hat. $225 for food, $65 for car expenses, and
                                                      $50 for entertainment. Find the total
                                                      amount budgeted for the three items each
                                                      month.   2. _____

3. The attendance at the Thursday afternoon   4. A hospital's emergency staff treated 83   3. _____
    lecture was 2592, and the attendance at the   people on Friday, 92 people on Saturday,
    Friday afternoon lecture was 643. Find the   and 64 people on Sunday. How many
    total attendance for the two lectures.   people did the emergency room staff treat
                                                    from Friday to Sunday?   4. _____

5. A real estate broker received commissions 6. During the first 4 months of the year, an   5. _____
    of $4650, $3920, $4425, and $2575 during   appliance store sold 675 toasters. The store
    a four month period. Find the total income   sold 127 toasters in May and 87 in June.
    from commissions for the four months.   How many toasters were sold during the
                                                    first six months of the year?   6. _____

7. You had a balance of $753 in your   8. You are leaving for a four-day vacation.   7. _____
    checking account before making deposits   The odometer on your car reads 61,795
    of $158, $269, and $374. What is your   miles. You plan to drive 185 miles the first
    new checking account balance?   day, 209 miles the second day, and 174
                                                     miles the third day. What will be your   8. _____
                                                     odometer reading at the end of the trip?

9. The new homeowner had the following   10. A software company made profits of   9. _____
    monthly expenses: mortgage–$900, $7,420,572, $1,764,025, and $6,871,429
    utilities–$194, insurance–$92, food–$526,   during its first three years. Find the
    and transportation–$78. Find the total costs   software company's total profit for the
    for the month.   three years.   10. _____

Name   Score

Subtract.

1.   9
      $- 4$

2.   6
      $- 3$

3.   7
      $- 6$

4.   25
     $- 10$

5.   58
     $- 47$

6.   98
     $- 37$

7.   179
    $- 84$

8.   453
    $- 53$

9.   164
    $- 93$

10.   691
     $- 130$

11.   889
     $- 667$

12.   905
     $- 602$

13.   8714
    $- 301$

14.   1539
    $- 722$

15.   2408
    $- 204$

16.   3215
    $- 2100$

17.   4976
    $- 3724$

18.   5341
    $- 3210$

19. $29 - 8$

20. $14 - 6$

21. $863 - 42$

22. $827 - 16$

23. $7538 - 532$

24. $1249 - 828$

25. $9527 - 7416$

26. $7884 - 1733$

1. _____
2. _____
3. _____
4. _____
5. _____
6. _____
7. _____
8. _____
9. _____
10. _____
11. _____
12. _____
13. _____
14. _____
15. _____
16. _____
17. _____
18. _____
19. _____
20. _____
21. _____
22. _____
23. _____
24. _____
25. _____
26. _____

Name   Score

Subtract.

1. 63 − 19	**2.** 84 − 26	**3.** 98 − 39	**1.** _____
			2. _____
			3. _____
4. 273 − 185	**5.** 432 − 378	**6.** 771 − 592	**4.** _____
			5. _____
			6. _____
7. 3645 − 376	**8.** 5094 − 695	**9.** 1419 − 453	**7.** _____
			8. _____
			9. _____
10. 6420 − 3990	**11.** 8311 − 7499	**12.** 4936 − 1117	**10.** _____
			11. _____
			12. _____
13. 22,653 − 18,734	**14.** 53,417 − 26,718	**15.** 79,600 − 35,752	**13.** _____
			14. _____
			15. _____
16. 83,602 − 64,575	**17.** 248,000 − 96,729	**18.** 900,721 − 546,847	**16.** _____
			17. _____
			18. _____
19. 421 − 46	**20.** 725 − 88		**19.** _____
			20. _____
21. 5303 − 627	**22.** 8263 − 782		**21.** _____
			22. _____
23. 30,736 − 5947	**24.** 64,057 − 7316		**23.** _____
			24. _____
25. 56,322 − 29,415	**26.** 94,032 − 78,450		**25.** _____
			26. _____

Name   Score

Solve.

1. How much change will a customer receive 2. The down payment on a boat costing   1. _____
    after paying for a $27 purchase with a $50 $9655 is $1931. Find the amount that
    bill?   remains to be paid.
                                                                                                2. _____

3. You drove a car 31,672 miles in a three- 4. After a trip of 649 miles, the odometer of   3. _____
    year period. You drove 9670 miles the first   your car read 54,456 miles. What was the
    year and 11,426 miles the second year.   odometer reading at the beginning of your
    How many miles did you drive the third   trip?
    year?   4. _____

5. Your monthly food budget is $380. How   6. You had a bank balance of $932. You then   5. _____
    much is left in the food budget after   wrote checks for $183, $74, and $25. Find
    spending $169 on groceries?   the new bank balance.
                                                                                                6. _____

7. A lab technician receives a total salary of 8. A public relations executive has an   7. _____
    $4650 per month. Deductions from the   expense account of $1100. The amount
    check are $1068 for taxes, $278 for social   already spent includes $238 for
    security, and $84 for insurance. Find the lab transportation, $130 for food, and $366 for
    technician's take-home pay.   lodging. Find the balance remaining in the 8. _____
                                                   expense account.

9. Your monthly budget for household   10. How much larger is Texas than Wyoming?   9. _____
    expenses is $800. After $238 is spent for   Texas is 266,873 square miles in area, and
    food, $129 for clothes, and $48 for   Wyoming is 97,809 square miles in area.
    entertainment, how much is left in the   10. _____
    budget?

Name   Score

Multiply.

1.   9
    × 7
	2. 0
	    × 6
		3. 5
		    × 4

1. _____

2. _____

3. _____

4.   6
    × 8
	5. 5
	    × 3
		6. 6
		    × 6

4. _____

5. _____

6. _____

7.   69
   × 3
	8. 24
	   × 7
		9. 71
		   × 6

7. _____

8. _____

9. _____

10.   49
   × 5
	11. 76
	   × 9
		12. 38
		   × 4

10. _____

11. _____

12. _____

13.   158
   × 2
	14. 649
	   × 8
		15. 273
		   × 6

13. _____

14. _____

15. _____

16.   845
   × 5
	17. 555
	   × 7
		18. 841
		   × 3

16. _____

17. _____

18. _____

19.   1136
   × 7
	20. 4721
	   × 6
		21. 7894
		   × 9

19. _____

20. _____

21. _____

22.   6543
   × 4
	23. 2199
	   × 8
		24. 3724
		   × 5

22. _____

23. _____

24. _____

25.   17,234
   × 3
	26. 51,990
	   × 7
		27. 45,616
		   × 9

25. _____

26. _____

27. _____

Name   Score

Multiply.

1.   14   2.   30   3.   75   1. _____
     × 28   × 62   × 42
                                                          2. _____

                                                          3. _____

4.   59   5.   39   6.   83   4. _____
     × 11   × 45   × 96
                                                          5. _____

                                                          6. _____

7.   281   8.   495   9.   845   7. _____
     × 64   × 37   × 56
                                                          8. _____

                                                          9. _____

10.   856   11.   625   12.   399   10. _____
     × 71   × 18   × 57
                                                          11. _____

                                                          12. _____

13. 7815   14. 5146   15. 9488   13. _____
     × 26   × 83   × 77
                                                          14. _____

                                                          15. _____

16. 3012   17. 8400   18. 3289   16. _____
     × 61   × 53   × 32
                                                          17. _____

                                                          18. _____

19.   391   20.   724   21.   298   19. _____
     × 465   × 831   × 665
                                                          20. _____

                                                          21. _____

22. 2911   23. 5673   24. 3485   22. _____
     × 643   × 394   × 865
                                                          23. _____

                                                          24. _____

25. 3600   26. 6412   27. 8923   25. _____
     × 240   × 180   × 336
                                                          26. _____

                                                          27. _____

11

Name _____   Score _____

Solve.

1. The Environmental Protection Agency (EPA) estimates that a motorcycles gets 38 miles on one gallon of gas. How many miles could it get on 6 gallons of gas?

2. The truck driver drove at a constant speed of 53 miles per hour for 6 hours. Find the distance the truck driver traveled.

1. _____

2. _____

3. A librarian catalogued 27 shelves of books. Each shelf held 32 books. How many books did the librarian catalogue?

4. An investor receives a check for $394 each month. How much will the investor receive over a 24-month period?

3. _____

4. _____

5. A mechanic has a car payment of $254 each month. What is the total of car payments over a 12-month period?

6. A data-entry operator earns $494 for working a 40-hour week. Last week the operator worked an additional 5 hours at $18 per hour. Find the data-entry operator's total pay for last week's work.

5. _____

6. _____

7. It takes approximately 709 hours for the moon to make one revolution around Earth. How many hours would it take the moon to make 12 revolutions around Earth?

8. A baker can buy 1000 pounds of flour for $150 and one 100-pound bag of sugar for $32. The baker orders 1000 pounds of flour and fifteen 100-pound bags of sugar. What is the total cost of the order?

7. _____

8. _____

9. A gasoline storage tank contains 65,000 gallons of gasoline. A valve is opened which lets out 40 gallons each minute. How many gallons remain in the tank after 45 minutes?

10. The average annual salary of a publishing company's employees is $51,280. If there are 156 people employed at the company, what is the total amount spent annually on salaries?

9. _____

10. _____

12

Name _____ Score _____

Divide.

1. $3\overline{)6}$

2. $2\overline{)4}$

3. $9\overline{)9}$

4. $7\overline{)84}$

5. $6\overline{)42}$

6. $4\overline{)16}$

7. $5\overline{)95}$

8. $9\overline{)72}$

9. $3\overline{)33}$

10. $4\overline{)540}$

11. $5\overline{)625}$

12. $8\overline{)656}$

13. $7\overline{)343}$

14. $3\overline{)1575}$

15. $5\overline{)2280}$

16. $6\overline{)3162}$

17. $4\overline{)1596}$

18. $7\overline{)38,927}$

19. $5\overline{)57,395}$

20. $6\overline{)31,404}$

21. $8\overline{)61,112}$

1. _____

2. _____

3. _____

4. _____

5. _____

6. _____

7. _____

8. _____

9. _____

10. _____

11. _____

12. _____

13. _____

14. _____

15. _____

16. _____

17. _____

18. _____

19. _____

20. _____

21. _____

Name   Score

Divide.

1. $3\overline{)7}$ 2. $2\overline{)9}$ 3. $5\overline{)6}$

4. $6\overline{)29}$ 5. $3\overline{)47}$ 6. $5\overline{)61}$

7. $4\overline{)73}$ 8. $7\overline{)48}$ 9. $9\overline{)40}$

10. $4\overline{)693}$ 11. $7\overline{)355}$ 12. $6\overline{)890}$

13. $5\overline{)269}$ 14. $3\overline{)1178}$ 15. $5\overline{)4957}$

16. $9\overline{)6234}$ 17. $4\overline{)5913}$ 18. $5\overline{)37,234}$

19. $3\overline{)24,652}$ 20. $4\overline{)59,403}$ 21. $8\overline{)72,641}$

1. _____
2. _____
3. _____
4. _____
5. _____
6. _____
7. _____
8. _____
9. _____
10. _____
11. _____
12. _____
13. _____
14. _____
15. _____
16. _____
17. _____
18. _____
19. _____
20. _____
21. _____

Name

Score

Divide.

1. $23\overline{)94}$

2. $36\overline{)76}$

3. $52\overline{)83}$

4. $73\overline{)374}$

5. $21\overline{)147}$

6. $48\overline{)598}$

7. $53\overline{)274}$

8. $37\overline{)4762}$

9. $77\overline{)7941}$

10. $41\overline{)5913}$

11. $63\overline{)7623}$

12. $55\overline{)4418}$

13. $18\overline{)1536}$

14. $86\overline{)6393}$

15. $45\overline{)8398}$

16. $98\overline{)6010}$

17. $62\overline{)4335}$

18. $92\overline{)54,392}$

19. $48\overline{)38,120}$

20. $799\overline{)66,427}$

21. $243\overline{)19,197}$

1.   _____

2.   _____

3.   _____

4.   _____

5.   _____

6.   _____

7.   _____

8.   _____

9.   _____

10. _____

11. _____

12. _____

13. _____

14. _____

15. _____

16. _____

17. _____

18. _____

19. _____

20. _____

21. _____

Name _____   Score _____

Solve.

1. A farmer ships 120,000 bushels of corn in 8 railroad cars. Find the amount of corn shipped in each car, assuming each car holds the same amount.

2. A shipment of 8460 diodes requires testing. The diodes are divided equally among 15 employees. How many diodes must each employee test?

1. _____

2. _____

3. A lottery prize of $737,000 is divided equally among 4 winners. What amount does each winner receive?

4. The new movie premiered at 14 theatres last Friday. If 2240 people attended the premiere and they were distributed equally among the 14 theatres, how many people attended each theatre?

3. _____

4. _____

5. The total cost of a car, including finance charges, is $7632. This amount is to be repaid in 36 equal monthly payments. What is the amount of each payment?

6. A management consultant received a check for $1755 for 45 hours of work. What is the consultant's hourly wage?

5. _____

6. _____

7. A student obtains a no-interest loan of $4600 per year for three years. After that time the student must pay off the loan in equal monthly payments for a period of 120 months. What is the amount of the student's monthly payments?

8. A consumer makes a down payment of $4516 on a video entertainment center costing $6724. The balance is to be paid in 12 equal monthly payments. What is the payment for one month?

7. _____

8. _____

9. A fund-raising organization collected $1,128,193 in one year for 11 charities. If the charities share the money equally, how much will each one receive?

10. A tannery produces and packages 320 briefcases each hour. Ten briefcases are put in each package for shipment. How many packages of briefcases can be produced in 8 hours?

9. _____

10. _____

16

Name   Score

Write the number in exponential notation.

1. $4 \cdot 4 \cdot 4 \cdot 4$

2. $8 \cdot 8 \cdot 8 \cdot 8 \cdot 8 \cdot 8$

3. $3 \cdot 3 \cdot 3 \cdot 3 \cdot 4 \cdot 4$

4. $5 \cdot 5 \cdot 5 \cdot 5 \cdot 7 \cdot 7 \cdot 7$

5. $2 \cdot 6 \cdot 6 \cdot 6 \cdot 6 \cdot 6 \cdot 6 \cdot 6$

6. $6 \cdot 10 \cdot 10 \cdot 10 \cdot 10$

7. $2 \cdot 2 \cdot 2 \cdot 3 \cdot 3 \cdot 3 \cdot 3 \cdot 7 \cdot 7$

8. $5 \cdot 6 \cdot 7 \cdot 7 \cdot 8 \cdot 8 \cdot 8$

9. $4 \cdot 4 \cdot 5 \cdot 5 \cdot 5 \cdot 6 \cdot 6 \cdot 6 \cdot 7$

10. $7 \cdot 7 \cdot 7 \cdot 15 \cdot 15 \cdot 19 \cdot 19$

1. _____
2. _____
3. _____
4. _____
5. _____
6. _____
7. _____
8. _____
9. _____
10. _____

Simplify.

11. 2^4

12. 3^3

13. 4^3

14. $2^4 \cdot 3^5$

15. $4^2 \cdot 5^3$

16. $7^2 \cdot 8^3$

17. $0^5 \cdot 3^2 \cdot 6^4$

18. $2 \cdot 4^2 \cdot 10$

19. $5^2 \cdot 10^2 \cdot 15$

20. $3 \cdot 10^2 \cdot 7^3$

21. $2^3 \cdot 3^3 \cdot 4^3$

22. $7^2 \cdot 10 \cdot 3^4$

23. $9^2 \cdot 2^3 \cdot 6^2$

24. $5^3 \cdot 0^4 \cdot 8^3$

25. $5^2 \cdot 2^6 \cdot 9$

11. _____
12. _____
13. _____
14. _____
15. _____
16. _____
17. _____
18. _____
19. _____
20. _____
21. _____
22. _____
23. _____
24. _____
25. _____

Name   Score

Simplify by using the Order of Operations Agreement.

1. $8 - 2 + 6$ **2.** $9 - 3 + 5$ **3.** $7 + 4 \cdot 3$ **1.** _____

                                                                                        2. _____

                                                                                        3. _____

4. $3 \cdot 3 - 9$ **5.** $10 - 4 \div 2$ **6.** $8 + 3 - 6$ **4.** _____

                                                                                        5. _____

                                                                                        6. _____

7. $4^2 - 10$ **8.** $3(1 + 5) - 7$ **9.** $17 - 3^2$ **7.** _____

                                                                                        8. _____

                                                                                        9. _____

10. $8 \cdot (7 + 3) \div 8$ **11.** $7 \cdot 3^2 + 16$ **12.** $2^2 - 2(12 \div 6)$ **10.** _____

                                                                                        11. _____

                                                                                        12. _____

13. $13 + (9 - 7) \cdot 5$ **14.** $20 - 2 \cdot 3^2$ **15.** $4^2 + 6 \cdot (2 - 1)$ **13.** _____

                                                                                        14. _____

                                                                                        15. _____

16. $2^4 + 7 \cdot (5 - 5)$ **17.** $3^2 \cdot 4 + 6 \cdot 2^3$ **18.** $8 \cdot 2 - 3^2$ **16.** _____

                                                                                        17. _____

                                                                                        18. _____

19. $17 - 3 \cdot 5$ **20.** $14 + 4 \cdot 6$ **21.** $3 \cdot (8 - 7) + 10$ **19.** _____

                                                                                        20. _____

                                                                                        21. _____

22. $11 - (11 - 2) \div 3$ **23.** $7 \cdot (8 - 5) + 12$ **24.** $14 \div (3 + 4) \cdot 2$ **22.** _____

                                                                                        23. _____

                                                                                        24. _____

25. $8 - 5 + 9 \cdot 2 \div 3$ **26.** $6 \cdot 4 \div 3 \div 2 + 1$ **27.** $10(2 + 3) \div 5$ **25.** _____

                                                                                        26. _____

                                                                                        27. _____

Name _____ Score _____

Find all the factors of the number.

1. 2   2. 14   3. 21

4. 15   5. 23   6. 40

7. 38   8. 60   9. 58

10. 62   11. 81   12. 51

13. 99   14. 85   15. 70

16. 88   17. 63   18. 35

19. 45   20. 78   21. 55

22. 114   23. 121   24. 117

25. 150   26. 175   27. 181

1. _____

2. _____

3. _____

4. _____

5. _____

6. _____

7. _____

8. _____

9. _____

10. _____

11. _____

12. _____

13. _____

14. _____

15. _____

16. _____

17. _____

18. _____

19. _____

20. _____

21. _____

22. _____

23. _____

24. _____

25. _____

26. _____

27. _____

Name   Score

Find the prime factorization.

1. 8	**2.** 30	**3.** 53	**1.** _____
			2. _____
			3. _____
4. 10	**5.** 32	**6.** 64	**4.** _____
			5. _____
			6. _____
7. 11	**8.** 20	**9.** 82	**7.** _____
			8. _____
			9. _____
10. 35	**11.** 44	**12.** 69	**10.** _____
			11. _____
			12. _____
13. 72	**14.** 88	**15.** 94	**13.** _____
			14. _____
			15. _____
16. 60	**17.** 77	**18.** 100	**16.** _____
			17. _____
			18. _____
19. 104	**20.** 112	**21.** 124	**19.** _____
			20. _____
			21. _____
22. 130	**23.** 155	**24.** 200	**22.** _____
			23. _____
			24. _____
25. 315	**26.** 500	**27.** 260	**25.** _____
			26. _____
			27. _____

Name   Score

Find the LCM.

1. 3, 4	**2.** 3, 7	**3.** 6, 9	**1.** _____
			2. _____
			3. _____
4. 8, 10	**5.** 4, 8	**6.** 9, 12	**4.** _____
			5. _____
			6. _____
7. 4, 9	**8.** 6, 15	**9.** 16, 24	**7.** _____
			8. _____
			9. _____
10. 15, 25	**11.** 28, 32	**12.** 4, 18	**10.** _____
			11. _____
			12. _____
13. 72, 108	**14.** 84, 126	**15.** 32, 128	**13.** _____
			14. _____
			15. _____
16. 3, 7, 9	**17.** 6, 12, 27	**18.** 3, 7, 11	**16.** _____
			17. _____
			18. _____
19. 9, 12, 24	**20.** 10, 25, 40	**21.** 4, 7, 21	**19.** _____
			20. _____
			21. _____
22. 2, 7, 11	**23.** 28, 32, 56	**24.** 16, 20, 40	**22.** _____
			23. _____
			24. _____
25. 8, 27, 36	**26.** 6, 12, 18	**27.** 2, 16, 32	**25.** _____
			26. _____
			27. _____

Name   Score

Find the GCF.

1. 3, 7   **2.** 3, 6   **3.** 9, 16   **1.** _____

                                                                             2. _____

                                                                             3. _____

4. 8, 18   **5.** 10, 15   **6.** 30, 65   **4.** _____

                                                                             5. _____

                                                                             6. _____

7. 15, 30   **8.** 36, 56   **9.** 18, 27   **7.** _____

                                                                             8. _____

                                                                             9. _____

10. 21, 35   **11.** 15, 20   **12.** 30, 50   **10.** _____

                                                                             11. _____

                                                                             12. _____

13. 48, 64   **14.** 39, 52   **15.** 37, 67   **13.** _____

                                                                             14. _____

                                                                             15. _____

16. 4, 8, 10   **17.** 3, 5, 7   **18.** 3, 9, 12   **16.** _____

                                                                             17. _____

                                                                             18. _____

19. 5, 11, 13   **20.** 10, 25, 30   **21.** 16, 40, 80   **19.** _____

                                                                             20. _____

                                                                             21. _____

22. 16, 20, 32   **23.** 24, 32, 40   **24.** 18, 27, 81   **22.** _____

                                                                             23. _____

                                                                             24. _____

25. 28, 44, 56   **26.** 17, 68, 85   **27.** 30, 75, 150   **25.** _____

                                                                             26. _____

                                                                             27. _____

Name _____ Score _____

Express the shaded portion of the circle as a fraction.

1.

2.

3.

4.

1. _____

2. _____

3. _____

4. _____

Express the shaded portion of the circles as a mixed number.

5.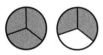

6.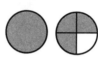

7.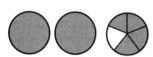

8.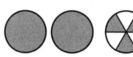

9.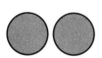

10.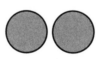

5. _____

6. _____

7. _____

8. _____

9. _____

10. _____

Express the shaded portion of the circles as an improper fraction.

11.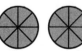

12.

13.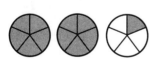

14.

11. _____

12. _____

13. _____

14. _____

Name   Score

Write the improper fraction as a mixed number or whole number.

1. $\dfrac{11}{3}$

2. $\dfrac{30}{5}$

3. $\dfrac{17}{9}$

4. $\dfrac{9}{2}$

5. $\dfrac{24}{9}$

6. $\dfrac{19}{4}$

7. $\dfrac{36}{12}$

8. $\dfrac{11}{6}$

9. $\dfrac{8}{8}$

10. $\dfrac{64}{8}$

11. $\dfrac{14}{1}$

12. $\dfrac{70}{14}$

1. _____

2. _____

3. _____

4. _____

5. _____

6. _____

7. _____

8. _____

9. _____

10. _____

11. _____

12. _____

Write the mixed number as an improper fraction.

13. $2\dfrac{1}{5}$

14. $7\dfrac{2}{3}$

15. $4\dfrac{7}{9}$

16. $2\dfrac{7}{8}$

17. $5\dfrac{2}{7}$

18. $6\dfrac{3}{5}$

19. $10\dfrac{3}{4}$

20. $9\dfrac{7}{10}$

21. $12\dfrac{5}{6}$

22. $7\dfrac{13}{15}$

23. $11\dfrac{1}{3}$

24. $16\dfrac{3}{8}$

13. _____

14. _____

15. _____

16. _____

17. _____

18. _____

19. _____

20. _____

21. _____

22. _____

23. _____

24. _____

Name

Score

Build an equivalent fraction with the given denominator.

1. $\dfrac{2}{3} = \dfrac{}{39}$

2. $\dfrac{5}{6} = \dfrac{}{18}$

3. $\dfrac{4}{7} = \dfrac{}{56}$

4. $\dfrac{1}{5} = \dfrac{}{25}$

5. $\dfrac{3}{4} = \dfrac{}{28}$

6. $\dfrac{6}{10} = \dfrac{}{30}$

7. $\dfrac{1}{2} = \dfrac{}{30}$

8. $\dfrac{4}{5} = \dfrac{}{45}$

9. $\dfrac{2}{9} = \dfrac{}{54}$

10. $\dfrac{8}{12} = \dfrac{}{48}$

11. $\dfrac{11}{13} = \dfrac{}{65}$

12. $\dfrac{5}{10} = \dfrac{}{70}$

13. $\dfrac{6}{7} = \dfrac{}{84}$

14. $6 = \dfrac{}{9}$

15. $8 = \dfrac{}{15}$

16. $\dfrac{2}{4} = \dfrac{}{36}$

17. $\dfrac{1}{3} = \dfrac{}{102}$

18. $\dfrac{5}{9} = \dfrac{}{180}$

19. $\dfrac{10}{15} = \dfrac{}{90}$

20. $\dfrac{17}{20} = \dfrac{}{96}$

21. $\dfrac{4}{11} = \dfrac{}{121}$

22. $\dfrac{8}{20} = \dfrac{}{240}$

23. $\dfrac{15}{16} = \dfrac{}{336}$

24. $\dfrac{7}{33} = \dfrac{}{165}$

25. $\dfrac{5}{8} = \dfrac{}{312}$

26. $\dfrac{14}{19} = \dfrac{}{437}$

27. $\dfrac{21}{25} = \dfrac{}{1075}$

1. _____
2. _____
3. _____
4. _____
5. _____
6. _____
7. _____
8. _____
9. _____
10. _____
11. _____
12. _____
13. _____
14. _____
15. _____
16. _____
17. _____
18. _____
19. _____
20. _____
21. _____
22. _____
23. _____
24. _____
25. _____
26. _____
27. _____

Name _____   Score _____

Reduce the fraction to simplest form.

1. $\dfrac{8}{12}$ 2. $\dfrac{15}{25}$ 3. $\dfrac{2}{16}$

4. $\dfrac{28}{49}$ 5. $\dfrac{54}{81}$ 6. $\dfrac{40}{64}$

7. $\dfrac{75}{90}$ 8. $\dfrac{36}{27}$ 9. $\dfrac{0}{15}$

10. $\dfrac{60}{96}$ 11. $\dfrac{18}{36}$ 12. $\dfrac{7}{18}$

13. $\dfrac{25}{100}$ 14. $\dfrac{84}{144}$ 15. $\dfrac{39}{13}$

16. $\dfrac{169}{234}$ 17. $\dfrac{112}{126}$ 18. $\dfrac{59}{177}$

19. $\dfrac{85}{65}$ 20. $\dfrac{34}{238}$ 21. $\dfrac{16}{34}$

22. $\dfrac{104}{240}$ 23. $\dfrac{69}{150}$ 24. $\dfrac{26}{75}$

25. $\dfrac{112}{160}$ 26. $\dfrac{143}{182}$ 27. $\dfrac{92}{23}$

1. _____
2. _____
3. _____
4. _____
5. _____
6. _____
7. _____
8. _____
9. _____
10. _____
11. _____
12. _____
13. _____
14. _____
15. _____
16. _____
17. _____
18. _____
19. _____
20. _____
21. _____
22. _____
23. _____
24. _____
25. _____
26. _____
27. _____

Name _____ Score _____

Add.

1. $\dfrac{3}{6}+\dfrac{2}{6}$

2. $\dfrac{5}{10}+\dfrac{6}{10}$

3. $\dfrac{7}{19}+\dfrac{3}{19}$

4. $\dfrac{2}{7}+\dfrac{4}{7}$

5. $\dfrac{4}{8}+\dfrac{3}{8}$

6. $\dfrac{11}{15}+\dfrac{4}{15}$

7. $\dfrac{5}{7}+\dfrac{9}{7}$

8. $\dfrac{3}{14}+\dfrac{1}{14}$

9. $\dfrac{3}{5}+\dfrac{6}{5}$

10. $\dfrac{13}{17}+\dfrac{2}{17}$

11. $\dfrac{2}{4}+\dfrac{1}{4}$

12. $\dfrac{7}{12}+\dfrac{5}{12}$

13. $\dfrac{1}{3}+\dfrac{2}{3}+\dfrac{4}{3}$

14. $\dfrac{5}{9}+\dfrac{4}{9}+\dfrac{7}{9}$

15. $\dfrac{4}{11}+\dfrac{9}{11}+\dfrac{1}{11}$

16. $\dfrac{7}{8}+\dfrac{10}{8}+\dfrac{3}{8}$

17. $\dfrac{6}{12}+\dfrac{2}{12}+\dfrac{3}{12}$

18. $\dfrac{5}{6}+\dfrac{8}{6}+\dfrac{1}{6}$

19. $\dfrac{3}{15}+\dfrac{9}{15}+\dfrac{1}{15}$

20. $\dfrac{6}{10}+\dfrac{1}{10}+\dfrac{8}{10}$

21. $\dfrac{3}{4}+\dfrac{6}{4}+\dfrac{8}{4}$

22. $\dfrac{6}{5}+\dfrac{2}{5}+\dfrac{3}{5}$

23. $\dfrac{7}{14}+\dfrac{3}{14}+\dfrac{8}{14}$

24. $\dfrac{8}{16}+\dfrac{2}{16}+\dfrac{9}{16}$

25. $\dfrac{4}{13}+\dfrac{11}{13}+\dfrac{14}{13}$

26. $\dfrac{15}{17}+\dfrac{12}{17}+\dfrac{5}{17}$

27. $\dfrac{2}{9}+\dfrac{6}{9}+\dfrac{9}{9}$

1. _____
2. _____
3. _____
4. _____
5. _____
6. _____
7. _____
8. _____
9. _____
10. _____
11. _____
12. _____
13. _____
14. _____
15. _____
16. _____
17. _____
18. _____
19. _____
20. _____
21. _____
22. _____
23. _____
24. _____
25. _____
26. _____
27. _____

Name _____   Score _____

Add.

1. $\dfrac{1}{4}+\dfrac{5}{6}$

2. $\dfrac{4}{15}+\dfrac{5}{9}$

3. $\dfrac{2}{3}+\dfrac{7}{8}$

4. $\dfrac{3}{4}+\dfrac{11}{16}$

5. $\dfrac{7}{9}+\dfrac{10}{12}$

6. $\dfrac{5}{6}+\dfrac{3}{8}$

7. $\dfrac{13}{14}+\dfrac{15}{18}$

8. $\dfrac{3}{14}+\dfrac{17}{21}$

9. $\dfrac{9}{10}+\dfrac{10}{16}$

10. $\dfrac{4}{16}+\dfrac{35}{40}$

11. $\dfrac{7}{12}+\dfrac{4}{8}$

12. $\dfrac{12}{15}+\dfrac{19}{20}$

13. $\dfrac{1}{2}+\dfrac{1}{4}+\dfrac{1}{6}$

14. $\dfrac{2}{5}+\dfrac{7}{10}+\dfrac{7}{15}$

15. $\dfrac{2}{3}+\dfrac{3}{7}+\dfrac{18}{21}$

16. $\dfrac{1}{4}+\dfrac{1}{3}+\dfrac{8}{9}$

17. $\dfrac{1}{2}+\dfrac{5}{8}+\dfrac{10}{12}$

18. $\dfrac{3}{5}+\dfrac{6}{7}+\dfrac{5}{9}$

19. $\dfrac{9}{12}+\dfrac{2}{4}+\dfrac{5}{16}$

20. $\dfrac{2}{3}+\dfrac{7}{9}+\dfrac{7}{10}$

21. $\dfrac{4}{5}+\dfrac{1}{6}+\dfrac{15}{18}$

22. $\dfrac{1}{2}+\dfrac{6}{7}+\dfrac{4}{8}$

23. $\dfrac{2}{3}+\dfrac{4}{6}+\dfrac{17}{18}$

24. $\dfrac{3}{4}+\dfrac{5}{7}+\dfrac{13}{14}$

25. $\dfrac{3}{6}+\dfrac{1}{8}+\dfrac{7}{10}$

26. $\dfrac{1}{5}+\dfrac{1}{11}+\dfrac{1}{15}$

27. $\dfrac{5}{6}+\dfrac{15}{24}+\dfrac{7}{8}$

1. _____
2. _____
3. _____
4. _____
5. _____
6. _____
7. _____
8. _____
9. _____
10. _____
11. _____
12. _____
13. _____
14. _____
15. _____
16. _____
17. _____
18. _____
19. _____
20. _____
21. _____
22. _____
23. _____
24. _____
25. _____
26. _____
27. _____

Name _____   Score _____

Add.

1. $3\frac{4}{9}$

    $+\ 2\frac{2}{3}$

2. $4\frac{2}{3}$

    $+\ 4\frac{5}{6}$

3. $5\frac{4}{7}$

    $+\ 7\frac{3}{4}$

4. 6

    $+\ 11\frac{7}{12}$

5. $8\frac{6}{14}$

    $+\ 3\frac{2}{8}$

6. $1\frac{4}{9}$

    $+\ 9\frac{11}{15}$

7. $6\frac{1}{2}+5\frac{2}{3}$

8. $7\frac{5}{6}+2\frac{13}{15}$

9. $4\frac{3}{5}+6\frac{4}{7}$

10. $1\frac{4}{9}+11\frac{15}{18}$

11. $3\frac{1}{4}+7\frac{1}{5}$

12. $18\frac{5}{8}+10\frac{9}{14}$

13. $5\frac{7}{10}+25\frac{4}{15}$

14. $9\frac{5}{6}+12\frac{1}{9}$

15. $3\frac{3}{7}+4\frac{7}{8}$

16. $8\frac{9}{10}+5\frac{11}{12}$

17. $15\frac{5}{11}+30\frac{2}{4}$

18. $21\frac{3}{5}+6\frac{5}{12}$

19. $3\frac{1}{3}+2\frac{1}{2}+9\frac{3}{4}$

20. $7\frac{4}{7}+1\frac{3}{14}+11\frac{2}{5}$

21. $6\frac{7}{9}+5\frac{11}{12}+10\frac{5}{10}$

22. $4\frac{5}{8}+8\frac{1}{2}+4\frac{7}{12}$

23. $2\frac{14}{15}+7\frac{17}{20}+1\frac{29}{30}$

24. $6\frac{15}{18}+9\frac{21}{30}+15\frac{11}{12}$

25. $1\frac{3}{4}+25\frac{3}{8}+6\frac{10}{12}$

26. $9\frac{3}{5}+5\frac{3}{5}+10\frac{3}{4}$

27. $2\frac{6}{7}+1\frac{1}{3}+14\frac{11}{21}$

1. _____
2. _____
3. _____
4. _____
5. _____
6. _____
7. _____
8. _____
9. _____
10. _____
11. _____
12. _____
13. _____
14. _____
15. _____
16. _____
17. _____
18. _____
19. _____
20. _____
21. _____
22. _____
23. _____
24. _____
25. _____
26. _____
27. _____

Name   Score

Solve.

1.   Over a two-year period, a child grew $4\frac{5}{8}$ inches. If the child grew $1\frac{1}{2}$ inches the first year, how many inches did the child grow during the second year?

2.   A wall that is $\frac{3}{4}$-inches thick is covered by a $\frac{5}{16}$-inch veneer. Find the total thickness after the never is installed.

1. _____

2. _____

3.   A carpenter build a header by nailing a $1\frac{1}{4}$-inch board to a $2\frac{5}{8}$-inch beam. Find the total thickness of the header.

4.   You bought stock in a publishing company for $18\frac{5}{8}$ ($18\frac{5}{8}$ per share). The price of the stock gained $4\frac{1}{2}$ ($4\frac{1}{2}$ per share) during a three-week period. Find the price of the stock at the end of the three weeks.

3. _____

4. _____

5.   Find the length of the shaft in the following diagram.

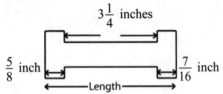

$3\frac{1}{4}$ inches

$\frac{5}{8}$ inch $\frac{7}{16}$ inch

Length

6.   A electrician works $2\frac{1}{4}$ hours of overtime on Monday, $2\frac{3}{4}$ hours on Tuesday, and $2\frac{1}{2}$ hours on Wednesday. Find the total number of hours of overtime worked during the three days.

5. _____

6. _____

7.   An artist places a $2\frac{7}{8}$-inch mat around a painting that is $16\frac{1}{2}$ inches long and $11\frac{3}{4}$ inches wide. Find the new dimensions of the picture.

8.   A shopper bought $\frac{1}{2}$ pound of cheese, $\frac{3}{4}$ pound of ham, $\frac{3}{4}$ pound of bologna, and $1\frac{1}{4}$ pounds of salami. How many pounds of cold cuts did the shopper buy?

7. _____

8. _____

9.   A recipe calls for $3\frac{1}{2}$ cups of rice, $2\frac{3}{4}$ cups of chopped celery, and $1\frac{1}{2}$ cups of sliced carrots. Find the total amount of rice, celery, and carrots needed for the recipe.

10. A plumber works $1\frac{1}{2}$ hours of overtime on Thursday and $2\frac{3}{4}$ hours on Friday. At a salary of $48 an hour, how much overtime pay does the plumber receive for the two days?

9. _____

10. _____

Name

Score

Subtract.

1. $\dfrac{7}{12}$ $-\dfrac{5}{12}$

2. $\dfrac{17}{24}$ $-\dfrac{7}{24}$

3. $\dfrac{13}{18}$ $-\dfrac{7}{18}$

4. $\dfrac{23}{30}$ $-\dfrac{7}{30}$

5. $\dfrac{14}{15}$ $-\dfrac{2}{15}$

6. $\dfrac{9}{28}$ $-\dfrac{2}{28}$

7. $\dfrac{16}{25}$ $-\dfrac{4}{25}$

8. $\dfrac{31}{40}$ $-\dfrac{19}{40}$

9. $\dfrac{21}{32}$ $-\dfrac{9}{32}$

10. $\dfrac{13}{20}$ $-\dfrac{3}{20}$

11. $\dfrac{8}{11}$ $-\dfrac{2}{11}$

12. $\dfrac{12}{23}$ $-\dfrac{4}{23}$

13. $\dfrac{43}{56}$ $-\dfrac{19}{56}$

14. $\dfrac{24}{27}$ $-\dfrac{10}{27}$

15. $\dfrac{5}{13}$ $-\dfrac{3}{13}$

16. $\dfrac{15}{16}$ $-\dfrac{9}{16}$

17. $\dfrac{11}{21}$ $-\dfrac{4}{21}$

18. $\dfrac{23}{26}$ $-\dfrac{5}{26}$

19. $\dfrac{7}{12}$ $-\dfrac{5}{12}$

20. $\dfrac{44}{45}$ $-\dfrac{4}{45}$

21. $\dfrac{14}{17}$ $-\dfrac{12}{17}$

22. $\dfrac{49}{60}$ $-\dfrac{7}{60}$

23. $\dfrac{13}{14}$ $-\dfrac{3}{14}$

24. $\dfrac{8}{35}$ $-\dfrac{4}{35}$

25. $\dfrac{14}{19}$ $-\dfrac{6}{19}$

26. $\dfrac{26}{29}$ $-\dfrac{15}{29}$

27. $\dfrac{15}{22}$ $-\dfrac{7}{22}$

1. _____
2. _____
3. _____
4. _____
5. _____
6. _____
7. _____
8. _____
9. _____
10. _____
11. _____
12. _____
13. _____
14. _____
15. _____
16. _____
17. _____
18. _____
19. _____
20. _____
21. _____
22. _____
23. _____
24. _____
25. _____
26. _____
27. _____

Name   Score

Subtract.

1.
$$\frac{3}{5}$$
$$-\frac{1}{4}$$

2.
$$\frac{14}{15}$$
$$-\frac{1}{6}$$

3.
$$\frac{11}{14}$$
$$-\frac{27}{42}$$

4.
$$\frac{13}{21}$$
$$-\frac{23}{49}$$

5.
$$\frac{7}{8}$$
$$-\frac{15}{32}$$

6.
$$\frac{16}{19}$$
$$-\frac{16}{57}$$

7.
$$\frac{22}{27}$$
$$-\frac{14}{45}$$

8.
$$\frac{33}{40}$$
$$-\frac{7}{16}$$

9.
$$\frac{1}{6}$$
$$-\frac{2}{13}$$

10.
$$\frac{26}{35}$$
$$-\frac{4}{15}$$

11.
$$\frac{1}{4}$$
$$-\frac{1}{10}$$

12.
$$\frac{17}{36}$$
$$-\frac{3}{20}$$

13.
$$\frac{25}{27}$$
$$-\frac{11}{18}$$

14.
$$\frac{7}{8}$$
$$-\frac{19}{24}$$

15.
$$\frac{9}{10}$$
$$-\frac{5}{12}$$

16.
$$\frac{25}{33}$$
$$-\frac{4}{9}$$

17.
$$\frac{29}{35}$$
$$-\frac{18}{25}$$

18.
$$\frac{5}{8}$$
$$-\frac{5}{18}$$

19.
$$\frac{14}{15}$$
$$-\frac{7}{12}$$

20.
$$\frac{6}{7}$$
$$-\frac{3}{5}$$

21.
$$\frac{9}{14}$$
$$-\frac{3}{10}$$

22.
$$\frac{51}{60}$$
$$-\frac{5}{12}$$

23.
$$\frac{23}{25}$$
$$-\frac{41}{50}$$

24.
$$\frac{19}{21}$$
$$-\frac{1}{6}$$

25.
$$\frac{17}{24}$$
$$-\frac{5}{9}$$

26.
$$\frac{23}{26}$$
$$-\frac{34}{39}$$

27.
$$\frac{5}{8}$$
$$-\frac{9}{20}$$

1. _____
2. _____
3. _____
4. _____
5. _____
6. _____
7. _____
8. _____
9. _____
10. _____
11. _____
12. _____
13. _____
14. _____
15. _____
16. _____
17. _____
18. _____
19. _____
20. _____
21. _____
22. _____
23. _____
24. _____
25. _____
26. _____
27. _____

Name _____ Score _____

Subtract.

1. $8\frac{9}{11}$
   $-4\frac{5}{11}$

2. $26\frac{15}{16}$
   $-11\frac{11}{16}$

3. $59\frac{19}{24}$
   $-18\frac{11}{24}$

4. $15\frac{15}{26}$
   -6

5. 12
   $-7\frac{15}{16}$

6. $17\frac{2}{5}$
   $-9\frac{4}{5}$

7. 44
   $-25\frac{4}{7}$

8. $36\frac{5}{14}$
   $-14\frac{9}{14}$

9. $27\frac{2}{5}$
   $-23\frac{4}{5}$

10. $65\frac{7}{9}$
    $-35\frac{5}{6}$

11. $89\frac{11}{15}$
    $-57\frac{17}{27}$

12. $52\frac{17}{35}$
    -29

13. $41\frac{7}{12}$
    $-17\frac{7}{16}$

14. 84
    $-48\frac{7}{12}$

15. $103\frac{3}{8}$
    $-54\frac{4}{7}$

16. $33\frac{8}{15}$
    $-19\frac{8}{9}$

17. $62\frac{17}{24}$
    $-28\frac{11}{16}$

18. $69\frac{19}{25}$
    $-60\frac{23}{25}$

19. 13
    $-7\frac{33}{40}$

20. $77\frac{32}{35}$
    $-38\frac{67}{70}$

21. $24\frac{5}{12}$
    $-15\frac{4}{9}$

22. $43\frac{16}{21}$
    $-34\frac{25}{42}$

23. $12\frac{2}{5}$
    $-9\frac{5}{6}$

24. $289\frac{9}{14}$
    $-163\frac{3}{8}$

25. $154\frac{7}{10}$
    $-78\frac{4}{5}$

26. $91\frac{37}{40}$
    $-38\frac{49}{60}$

27. $74\frac{8}{15}$
    $-57\frac{3}{20}$

1. _____
2. _____
3. _____
4. _____
5. _____
6. _____
7. _____
8. _____
9. _____
10. _____
11. _____
12. _____
13. _____
14. _____
15. _____
16. _____
17. _____
18. _____
19. _____
20. _____
21. _____
22. _____
23. _____
24. _____
25. _____
26. _____
27. _____

Name   Score

Solve.

1. A planer removes $\frac{1}{4}$ inch from a $\frac{5}{6}$-inch board. Find the resulting thickness of the board.

2. A $2\frac{2}{9}$–foot piece is cut from a 4-foot board. How much of the board is left?

1. _____

2. _____

3. You painted $\frac{3}{5}$ of your house today. How much of the paint job remains to be done?

4. In an athletic competition, the two best long jump attempts measured $23\frac{3}{4}$ feet and $25\frac{1}{6}$ feet. Find the difference between the two best jumps.

3. _____

4. _____

5. Find the missing dimension.

$8\frac{5}{6}$ feet

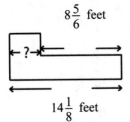

$14\frac{1}{8}$ feet

6. A plane trip from Boston to San Francisco takes $8\frac{1}{2}$ hours. After the plane is in the air to $5\frac{3}{4}$ hours, how much time remains before landing?

5. _____

6. _____

7. A three-day, $32\frac{1}{8}$-mile hike is planned. A hiker travels $10\frac{1}{5}$ miles the first day and $11\frac{3}{10}$ miles the second day. How many miles are left to travel on the third day?

8. For an upcoming role, an actor is put on a diet to lose 15 pounds. If $3\frac{1}{2}$ pounds are lost the first week and $2\frac{1}{4}$ pounds the second week, how many pounds must be lost to achieve the goal?

7. _____

8. _____

9. Two painters are staining a house. In one day, one painter stains $\frac{1}{5}$ of the house while the other stains $\frac{1}{4}$ of the house. How much of the job remains to be done?

10. A 10-mile race has 2 checkpoints. The first checkpoint is $4\frac{1}{2}$ miles from the starting point. The second checkpoint is $3\frac{5}{4}$ miles from the first checkpoint. How many miles is it from the second checkpoint to the finish line?

9. _____

10. _____

Name   Score

Multiply.

1. $\dfrac{4}{5} \times \dfrac{10}{13}$

2. $\dfrac{3}{4} \times \dfrac{8}{11}$

3. $\dfrac{4}{15} \times \dfrac{5}{9}$

4. $\dfrac{3}{10} \times \dfrac{5}{8}$

5. $\dfrac{5}{6} \times \dfrac{7}{11}$

6. $\dfrac{13}{18} \times \dfrac{1}{3}$

7. $\dfrac{4}{7} \times \dfrac{11}{16}$

8. $\dfrac{5}{9} \times \dfrac{5}{8}$

9. $\dfrac{5}{4} \times \dfrac{7}{10}$

10. $\dfrac{14}{15} \times \dfrac{7}{12}$

11. $\dfrac{5}{2} \times \dfrac{23}{20}$

12. $\dfrac{8}{15} \times \dfrac{6}{7}$

13. $\dfrac{9}{10} \times \dfrac{13}{18}$

14. $\dfrac{3}{7} \times \dfrac{5}{8}$

15. $\dfrac{12}{19} \times \dfrac{19}{6}$

16. $\dfrac{22}{14} \times \dfrac{16}{17}$

17. $\dfrac{21}{50} \times \dfrac{15}{24}$

18. $\dfrac{2}{5} \times \dfrac{15}{16}$

19. $\dfrac{7}{12} \times \dfrac{16}{9}$

20. $\dfrac{3}{8} \times \dfrac{10}{17}$

21. $\dfrac{6}{11} \times \dfrac{1}{4}$

22. $\dfrac{5}{6} \times \dfrac{9}{14}$

23. $\dfrac{1}{3} \times \dfrac{9}{10}$

24. $\dfrac{56}{85} \times \dfrac{51}{40}$

25. $\dfrac{9}{7} \times \dfrac{7}{9}$

26. $\dfrac{13}{66} \times \dfrac{11}{39}$

27. $\dfrac{6}{7} \times \dfrac{11}{13}$

1. _____
2. _____
3. _____
4. _____
5. _____
6. _____
7. _____
8. _____
9. _____
10. _____
11. _____
12. _____
13. _____
14. _____
15. _____
16. _____
17. _____
18. _____
19. _____
20. _____
21. _____
22. _____
23. _____
24. _____
25. _____
26. _____
27. _____

Name   Score

Multiply.

1. $4 \times \dfrac{7}{8}$

2. $7 \times \dfrac{2}{11}$

3. $7\dfrac{1}{2} \times \dfrac{4}{7}$

4. $\dfrac{2}{3} \times 3\dfrac{3}{4}$

5. $\dfrac{5}{6} \times 30$

6. $1\dfrac{4}{9} \times \dfrac{3}{10}$

7. $9 \times 3\dfrac{2}{3}$

8. $11\dfrac{1}{2} \times \dfrac{2}{13}$

9. $3\dfrac{4}{15} \times 3$

10. $\dfrac{4}{7} \times 2\dfrac{7}{12}$

11. $0 \times 3\dfrac{1}{6}$

12. $10 \times 5\dfrac{8}{15}$

13. $6\dfrac{3}{5} \times 8\dfrac{1}{6}$

14. $12\dfrac{3}{11} \times 7\dfrac{1}{3}$

15. $4\dfrac{5}{14} \times 15\dfrac{1}{2}$

16. $8\dfrac{3}{4} \times 6\dfrac{4}{5}$

17. $3\dfrac{5}{24} \times 12$

18. $2\dfrac{1}{7} \times 16\dfrac{4}{5}$

19. $8\dfrac{2}{15} \times 4\dfrac{7}{17}$

20. $1\dfrac{4}{9} \times 5\dfrac{1}{16}$

21. $9\dfrac{1}{3} \times 11\dfrac{5}{8}$

22. $7\dfrac{1}{2} \times 3\dfrac{9}{11}$

23. $19\dfrac{1}{4} \times 1\dfrac{5}{7}$

24. $4\dfrac{17}{18} \times 54$

25. $8\dfrac{4}{5} \times 14\dfrac{1}{6}$

26. $3\dfrac{3}{25} \times 2\dfrac{1}{2}$

27. $6\dfrac{1}{2} \times 9\dfrac{3}{13}$

1. _____

2. _____

3. _____

4. _____

5. _____

6. _____

7. _____

8. _____

9. _____

10. _____

11. _____

12. _____

13. _____

14. _____

15. _____

16. _____

17. _____

18. _____

19. _____

20. _____

21. _____

22. _____

23. _____

24. _____

25. _____

26. _____

27. _____

Name _____   Score _____

Solve.

1. An apprentice bricklayer earns $24 an hour. What are the bricklayer's total earnings after working $7\frac{1}{4}$ hours?

2. A sports car gets 21 miles on each gallon of gasoline. How many miles can the car travel on $5\frac{2}{3}$ gallons of gasoline?

3. A board is $8\frac{3}{4}$ feet long. One fourth of the board is cut off. What is the length of the piece cut off?

4. A plumber earns $320 for each day worked. What is the total of the plumber's earnings for working $4\frac{2}{5}$ days.

5. A family has an income of $3888 each month. The family spends $\frac{2}{9}$ of its income on rent. How much of the family's income (in dollars) is spent on rent each month?

6. A company budgets $\frac{1}{10}$ of its income each month for advertising. In June, the company had an income of $110,100. What is the amount budgeted for advertising in June?

7. A student read $\frac{2}{5}$ of a book containing 645 pages. How many pages did the student read?

8. A person can walk $3\frac{1}{4}$ miles in one hour. How many miles can the person walk in $1\frac{3}{4}$ hours?

9. An administrative assistant's gross weekly salary is $648. If $\frac{1}{4}$ of this amount is deducted for taxes, what is the administrative assistant's net weekly salary?

10. A sales representative has completed $\frac{3}{7}$ of a 1316-mile business trip. How many miles of the trip remain?

1. _____

2. _____

3. _____

4. _____

5. _____

6. _____

7. _____

8. _____

9. _____

10. _____

Name   Score

Divide.

1. $\dfrac{1}{9} \div \dfrac{2}{3}$

2. $\dfrac{5}{12} \div \dfrac{5}{16}$

3. $\dfrac{7}{10} \div \dfrac{14}{3}$

4. $\dfrac{3}{4} \div \dfrac{15}{6}$

5. $\dfrac{4}{11} \div \dfrac{12}{17}$

6. $3 \div \dfrac{9}{11}$

7. $\dfrac{4}{5} \div \dfrac{8}{5}$

8. $\dfrac{5}{24} \div \dfrac{5}{12}$

9. $\dfrac{10}{19} \div \dfrac{14}{19}$

10. $\dfrac{5}{9} \div \dfrac{2}{9}$

11. $\dfrac{16}{9} \div \dfrac{8}{3}$

12. $\dfrac{6}{11} \div \dfrac{3}{7}$

13. $0 \div \dfrac{1}{4}$

14. $\dfrac{9}{20} \div \dfrac{8}{55}$

15. $\dfrac{2}{15} \div \dfrac{7}{12}$

16. $\dfrac{9}{16} \div \dfrac{3}{28}$

17. $\dfrac{3}{4} \div \dfrac{15}{8}$

18. $\dfrac{7}{36} \div \dfrac{1}{8}$

19. $\dfrac{9}{20} \div \dfrac{11}{30}$

20. $\dfrac{14}{15} \div 7$

21. $\dfrac{5}{18} \div \dfrac{5}{9}$

22. $\dfrac{6}{18} \div \dfrac{12}{19}$

23. $\dfrac{4}{5} \div \dfrac{4}{5}$

24. $\dfrac{18}{35} \div \dfrac{3}{7}$

25. $\dfrac{1}{2} \div \dfrac{9}{8}$

26. $6 \div \dfrac{3}{8}$

27. $\dfrac{3}{7} \div \dfrac{9}{14}$

1. _____
2. _____
3. _____
4. _____
5. _____
6. _____
7. _____
8. _____
9. _____
10. _____
11. _____
12. _____
13. _____
14. _____
15. _____
16. _____
17. _____
18. _____
19. _____
20. _____
21. _____
22. _____
23. _____
24. _____
25. _____
26. _____
27. _____

Name _____ Score _____

Divide.

1. $\dfrac{3}{7} \div 3$

2. $8 \div \dfrac{16}{19}$

3. $24 \div \dfrac{4}{15}$

4. $4 \div 2\dfrac{2}{3}$

5. $\dfrac{4}{5} \div 2\dfrac{3}{4}$

6. $3\dfrac{3}{5} \div 9$

7. $1\dfrac{7}{12} \div \dfrac{7}{8}$

8. $21\dfrac{1}{4} \div 17$

9. $4\dfrac{3}{4} \div 3\dfrac{1}{3}$

10. $2\dfrac{3}{5} \div 2\dfrac{9}{10}$

11. $16\dfrac{3}{7} \div 1\dfrac{9}{14}$

12. $\dfrac{31}{35} \div 12\dfrac{2}{5}$

13. $15 \div 1\dfrac{1}{10}$

14. $18\dfrac{7}{16} \div 6\dfrac{3}{4}$

15. $30\dfrac{3}{8} \div 2\dfrac{1}{40}$

16. $5\dfrac{5}{12} \div 13\dfrac{13}{24}$

17. $\dfrac{3}{8} \div 8\dfrac{5}{8}$

18. $11\dfrac{1}{13} \div 48$

19. $9\dfrac{4}{8} \div 4\dfrac{9}{10}$

20. $18\dfrac{6}{22} \div 7\dfrac{1}{11}$

21. $20\dfrac{5}{9} \div 6\dfrac{2}{3}$

22. $\dfrac{25}{48} \div 15$

23. $3\dfrac{1}{2} \div 12\dfrac{11}{16}$

24. $4\dfrac{6}{7} \div 2\dfrac{1}{14}$

25. $9\dfrac{5}{11} \div 8\dfrac{2}{3}$

26. $17\dfrac{9}{14} \div \dfrac{13}{21}$

27. $10\dfrac{5}{18} \div 5\dfrac{5}{6}$

1. _____
2. _____
3. _____
4. _____
5. _____
6. _____
7. _____
8. _____
9. _____
10. _____
11. _____
12. _____
13. _____
14. _____
15. _____
16. _____
17. _____
18. _____
19. _____
20. _____
21. _____
22. _____
23. _____
24. _____
25. _____
26. _____
27. _____

Name　　　　　　　　　　　　　　　　　　　　　　　　　　　　Score

Solve.

1. An investor purchased a $3\frac{1}{4}$-ounce gold coin for $2028. What was the price for one ounce?

2. A car traveled 143 miles in $3\frac{1}{4}$ hours. What was the car's average speed in miles per hour?

3. A station wagon used $15\frac{3}{10}$ gallons of gasoline on a 306-mile trip. How many miles did this car travel on one gallon of gasoline?

4. A volunteer for the psychology experiment answered "yes" to 18 of the questions on one questionnaire. This was $\frac{3}{8}$ of the total number of questions. Find the total number of questions on the questionnaire.

5. If 55,000 people voted for the new city ordinance, and this was $\frac{5}{6}$ of the total number of registered voters in the city, how many registered voters are there?

6. A $2\frac{1}{2}$-grain precious metal ingot sold for $30. Find the price per grain of the precious metal.

7. A doll maker uses $2\frac{2}{3}$ yards of fabric to make a doll. How many dolls can be made with 32 yards of fabric?

8. A building contractor bought $8\frac{1}{4}$ acres of land for $396,000. What was the cost for each acre?

9. A 14-foot piece of wood molding is cut into pieces $4\frac{1}{4}$ feet long. What is the length of the piece remaining after cutting as many pieces as possible?

10. Of the total number of students in the introductory mathematics class, $\frac{1}{3}$ were taking the course as a review and 82 students were taking the course for the first time. Find the total number of students in the mathematics class.

1. _____

2. _____

3. _____

4. _____

5. _____

6. _____

7. _____

8. _____

9. _____

10. _____

Name _____   Score _____

Place the correct symbol, < or >, between the two numbers.

1. $\dfrac{11}{17}$ $\dfrac{14}{17}$

2. $\dfrac{4}{5}$ $\dfrac{5}{9}$

3. $\dfrac{7}{10}$ $\dfrac{2}{3}$

4. $\dfrac{7}{12}$ $\dfrac{11}{15}$

5. $\dfrac{5}{7}$ $\dfrac{3}{4}$

6. $\dfrac{2}{3}$ $\dfrac{3}{5}$

7. $\dfrac{3}{10}$ $\dfrac{1}{6}$

8. $\dfrac{7}{9}$ $\dfrac{9}{14}$

9. $\dfrac{4}{11}$ $\dfrac{1}{2}$

10. $\dfrac{1}{4}$ $\dfrac{4}{15}$

11. $\dfrac{13}{20}$ $\dfrac{5}{7}$

12. $\dfrac{8}{13}$ $\dfrac{11}{18}$

13. $\dfrac{19}{24}$ $\dfrac{25}{36}$

14. $\dfrac{8}{15}$ $\dfrac{23}{35}$

15. $\dfrac{5}{9}$ $\dfrac{3}{5}$

16. $\dfrac{5}{22}$ $\dfrac{3}{8}$

17. $\dfrac{1}{4}$ $\dfrac{5}{26}$

18. $\dfrac{5}{12}$ $\dfrac{4}{9}$

19. $\dfrac{9}{16}$ $\dfrac{10}{17}$

20. $\dfrac{19}{22}$ $\dfrac{39}{46}$

21. $\dfrac{23}{30}$ $\dfrac{17}{20}$

22. $\dfrac{5}{6}$ $\dfrac{3}{4}$

23. $\dfrac{11}{14}$ $\dfrac{15}{19}$

24. $\dfrac{7}{24}$ $\dfrac{8}{15}$

25. $\dfrac{4}{5}$ $\dfrac{16}{21}$

26. $\dfrac{7}{15}$ $\dfrac{5}{8}$

27. $\dfrac{21}{25}$ $\dfrac{27}{35}$

1. _____
2. _____
3. _____
4. _____
5. _____
6. _____
7. _____
8. _____
9. _____
10. _____
11. _____
12. _____
13. _____
14. _____
15. _____
16. _____
17. _____
18. _____
19. _____
20. _____
21. _____
22. _____
23. _____
24. _____
25. _____
26. _____
27. _____

Name   Score

Simplify.

1. $\left(\dfrac{5}{11}\right)^2$ 2. $\left(\dfrac{3}{7}\right)^2$ 3. $\left(\dfrac{5}{8}\right)^2$

4. $\left(\dfrac{3}{5}\right)^2\left(\dfrac{5}{7}\right)$ 5. $\left(\dfrac{3}{5}\right)\left(\dfrac{10}{21}\right)^2$ 6. $\left(\dfrac{2}{15}\right)^2\left(\dfrac{3}{4}\right)^2$

7. $\left(\dfrac{1}{2}\right)^2\left(\dfrac{4}{7}\right)$ 8. $\left(\dfrac{2}{21}\right)^2\left(\dfrac{3}{8}\right)$ 9. $\left(\dfrac{2}{9}\right)^4\left(\dfrac{3}{16}\right)^2$

10. $\left(\dfrac{1}{3}\right)^6\left(\dfrac{9}{11}\right)^2$ 11. $\left(\dfrac{5}{12}\right)^2\left(\dfrac{27}{50}\right)$ 12. $\left(\dfrac{4}{5}\right)^2\left(\dfrac{10}{19}\right)^2$

13. $\left(\dfrac{5}{27}\right)^2\left(\dfrac{3}{10}\right)^3$ 14. $\left(\dfrac{2}{9}\right)^3\left(\dfrac{3}{20}\right)^4$ 15. $\left(\dfrac{5}{63}\right)\left(\dfrac{7}{15}\right)^2$

16. $\left(\dfrac{8}{15}\right)\left(\dfrac{5}{6}\right)\left(\dfrac{3}{8}\right)^2$ 17. $\left(\dfrac{2}{5}\right)^2\left(\dfrac{5}{12}\right)^2\left(\dfrac{12}{17}\right)^2$ 18. $\left(\dfrac{2}{3}\right)^2\left(\dfrac{3}{4}\right)^2\left(\dfrac{4}{7}\right)$

19. $\left(\dfrac{1}{2}\right)^3\left(\dfrac{3}{8}\right)\left(\dfrac{8}{9}\right)^2$ 20. $4\cdot\left(\dfrac{5}{14}\right)\left(\dfrac{7}{10}\right)^2$ 21. $\left(\dfrac{3}{5}\right)^2\left(\dfrac{2}{3}\right)^3\left(\dfrac{5}{8}\right)^3$

22. $\left(\dfrac{3}{7}\right)^2\left(\dfrac{14}{17}\right)\cdot 17$ 23. $\left(\dfrac{5}{11}\right)\left(\dfrac{2}{9}\right)^2\left(\dfrac{3}{4}\right)^2$ 24. $\left(\dfrac{1}{6}\right)^2\left(\dfrac{1}{2}\right)^3\left(\dfrac{6}{7}\right)$

25. $\left(\dfrac{9}{16}\right)\left(\dfrac{2}{3}\right)^4\left(\dfrac{3}{13}\right)^3$ 26. $\left(\dfrac{4}{5}\right)^2\left(\dfrac{7}{11}\right)\left(\dfrac{5}{14}\right)^2$ 27. $13\cdot\left(\dfrac{1}{4}\right)^3\left(\dfrac{2}{13}\right)^2$

1. _____
2. _____
3. _____
4. _____
5. _____
6. _____
7. _____
8. _____
9. _____
10. _____
11. _____
12. _____
13. _____
14. _____
15. _____
16. _____
17. _____
18. _____
19. _____
20. _____
21. _____
22. _____
23. _____
24. _____
25. _____
26. _____
27. _____

Name _____   Score _____

Simplify using the Order of Operations Agreement.

1. $\dfrac{1}{4} + \dfrac{3}{7} - \dfrac{1}{6}$

2. $\dfrac{2}{3} - \dfrac{1}{5} + \dfrac{4}{9}$

3. $\dfrac{5}{8} + \dfrac{2}{9} \div \dfrac{8}{9}$

4. $\dfrac{4}{7} \div \dfrac{6}{11} + \dfrac{4}{5}$

5. $\dfrac{3}{4} \cdot \dfrac{5}{12} + \dfrac{9}{16}$

6. $\dfrac{1}{2} + \dfrac{4}{8} \cdot \dfrac{3}{10}$

7. $\left(\dfrac{5}{6}\right)^2 - \dfrac{2}{7}$

8. $\dfrac{7}{10} - \left(\dfrac{2}{3}\right)^3$

9. $\dfrac{5}{12} \cdot \left(\dfrac{4}{8} - \dfrac{8}{15}\right) + \dfrac{1}{3}$

10. $\dfrac{7}{8} \div \left(\dfrac{1}{4} + \dfrac{1}{10}\right) - \dfrac{7}{11}$

11. $\dfrac{3}{8} - \left(\dfrac{1}{2}\right)^3 + \dfrac{4}{9}$

12. $\dfrac{2}{5} + \left(\dfrac{2}{5}\right)^2 - \dfrac{4}{25}$

13. $\dfrac{1}{8} \div \left(\dfrac{1}{2}\right)^2 - \dfrac{1}{2}$

14. $\left(\dfrac{4}{7}\right)^2 \cdot \dfrac{3}{4} + \dfrac{11}{14}$

15. $\left(\dfrac{5}{8} + \dfrac{1}{4}\right) \cdot \dfrac{16}{21}$

16. $\dfrac{5}{6} \div \left(\dfrac{9}{10} - \dfrac{2}{15}\right)$

17. $\left(\dfrac{5}{9} + \dfrac{13}{18}\right) \div \left(\dfrac{2}{3}\right)^2$

18. $\left(\dfrac{1}{4}\right)^2 \cdot \left(\dfrac{7}{9} - \dfrac{1}{3}\right)$

19. $\dfrac{6}{7} \cdot \dfrac{14}{27} \div \dfrac{4}{9}$

20. $\left(\dfrac{1}{3}\right)^2 + \left(\dfrac{4}{5} - \dfrac{2}{3}\right) \div \dfrac{4}{5}$

21. $\left(\dfrac{4}{21}\right) \cdot \left(\dfrac{7}{8} + \dfrac{3}{4}\right) \div \dfrac{13}{14}$

22. $\dfrac{1}{6} + \left(\dfrac{1}{3} - \dfrac{3}{10}\right) \div \dfrac{7}{15}$

23. $\left(\dfrac{1}{2}\right)^3 - \left(\dfrac{2}{5}\right)\left(\dfrac{15}{22}\right) + \dfrac{1}{4}$

24. $\left(\dfrac{1}{3}\right)^2 + \left(\dfrac{5}{6} - \dfrac{3}{8}\right) \div \dfrac{5}{12}$

25. $\dfrac{8}{9} - \left(\dfrac{7}{10}\right)\left(\dfrac{2}{3}\right) \div \dfrac{4}{5}$

26. $\left(1\dfrac{1}{4} - \dfrac{2}{7} + \dfrac{1}{28}\right) \div \left(\dfrac{3}{13}\right)$

27. $\left(\dfrac{11}{12} - \dfrac{2}{3}\right) + \dfrac{15}{16} \div \left(\dfrac{1}{2}\right)^3$

1. _____

2. _____

3. _____

4. _____

5. _____

6. _____

7. _____

8. _____

9. _____

10. _____

11. _____

12. _____

13. _____

14. _____

15. _____

16. _____

17. _____

18. _____

19. _____

20. _____

21. _____

22. _____

23. _____

24. _____

25. _____

26. _____

27. _____

Name _____   Score _____

Write each decimal in words.

1. 0.39   2. 0.81   3. 2.007   1. _____

                                                            _____

                                                         2. _____

                                                            _____

                                                         3. _____

                                                            _____

4. 5.061   5. 15.4   6. 0.0086   4. _____

                                                            _____

                                                         5. _____

                                                            _____

                                                         6. _____

                                                            _____

7. 26.379   8. 514.3118   9. 1078.00002   7. _____

                                                            _____

                                                         8. _____

                                                            _____

                                                         9. _____

                                                            _____

Write each decimal in standard form.

10. Eight hundred thirty-four thousandths   11. Fifty-two millionths   10. _____

                                                                                11. _____

12. Six and one hundred one ten-thousandths 13. Eighty-seven and nine hundred six   12. _____
                                                 thousandths
                                                                                13. _____

14. Four hundred sixty-two and thirty-five   15. Six thousand fourteen and one thousand   14. _____
    thousandths   eight ten-thousandths
                                                                                15. _____

16. Twenty-five and seven thousand two   17. Ninety-one and seventeen ten-thousandths 16. _____
    hundred ninety-three hundred-thousandths
                                                                                17. _____

Name   Score

Round each decimal to the given place value.

1.   0.064 Tenths   2.   9.138 Tenths   1. _____

                                                                                2. _____

3.   26.349 Tenths   4.   96.4501 Tenths   3. _____

                                                                                4. _____

5.   65.34498 Hundredths   6.   13.01264 Hundredths   5. _____

                                                                                6. _____

7.   517.677 Hundredths   8.   792.246 Hundredths   7. _____

                                                                                8. _____

9.   2.09181 Thousandths   10. 6.27958 Thousandths   9. _____

                                                                                10. _____

11. 79.4625 Thousandths   12. 51.00439 Thousandths   11. _____

                                                                                12. _____

13. 0.04195 Ten-thousandths   14. 0.003642 Ten-thousandths   13. _____

                                                                                14. _____

15. 4.37628 Ten-thousandths   16. 16.111919 Ten-thousandths   15. _____

                                                                                16. _____

17. 0.249668 Hundred-thousandths   18. 0.009123 Hundred-thousandths   17. _____

                                                                                18. _____

19. 7.880102 Hundred-thousandths   20. 11.732405 Hundred-thousandths   19. _____

                                                                                20. _____

21. 1.49256 Nearest whole number   22. 3.60021 Nearest whole number   21. _____

                                                                                22. _____

23. 70.50648 Nearest whole number   24. 0.0045895 Millionths   23. _____

                                                                                24. _____

25. 0.10086438 Millionths   26. 2.11100649 Millionths   25. _____

                                                                                26. _____

Name   Score

Add.

1. $4.825 + 31.7894 + 168.67$ 2. $25.25 + 7.4418 + 18.5$

1. _____

2. _____

3. $6.841 + 54 + 59.3254$ 4. $85.0013 + 1.407 + 3.1114$

3. _____

4. _____

5. $39.1 + 2.4713 + 28.008$ 6. $5.066 + 18.751 + 1.091$

5. _____

6. _____

7. $6.421 + 52.118 + 3 + 0.0098$ 8. $4.46 + 2.3845 + 2.5 + 0.0231$

7. _____

8. _____

9. $0.0014 + 83.9 + 46 + 148.0908$ 10. $75.514 + 0.199 + 29 + 8.356$

9. _____

10. _____

11.
$$\begin{array}{r} 0.2 \\ + 1.09 \\ \hline \end{array}$$

12.
$$\begin{array}{r} 0.65 \\ + 0.9 \\ \hline \end{array}$$

13.
$$\begin{array}{r} 4.215 \\ + 6.8 \\ \hline \end{array}$$

11. _____

12. _____

13. _____

14.
$$\begin{array}{r} 3.217 \\ + 15.693 \\ \hline \end{array}$$

15.
$$\begin{array}{r} 12.093 \\ + 3.146 \\ \hline \end{array}$$

16.
$$\begin{array}{r} 32.22 \\ + 6.887 \\ \hline \end{array}$$

14. _____

15. _____

16. _____

17.
$$\begin{array}{r} 2.7156 \\ 45.08 \\ + 6.0406 \\ \hline \end{array}$$

18.
$$\begin{array}{r} 5.52 \\ 94.099 \\ + 7.2148 \\ \hline \end{array}$$

19.
$$\begin{array}{r} 11 \\ 77.29 \\ + 5.0531 \\ \hline \end{array}$$

17. _____

18. _____

19. _____

20.
$$\begin{array}{r} 97.01 \\ 8.456 \\ + 0.09 \\ \hline \end{array}$$

21.
$$\begin{array}{r} 42.056 \\ 15.6 \\ + 0.336 \\ \hline \end{array}$$

22.
$$\begin{array}{r} 5.271 \\ 67.013 \\ + 11.8 \\ \hline \end{array}$$

20. _____

21. _____

22. _____

23.
$$\begin{array}{r} 75.603 \\ 2.74 \\ 29 \\ + 53.008 \\ \hline \end{array}$$

24.
$$\begin{array}{r} 0.00051 \\ 6.8432 \\ 38.9121 \\ + 4.786 \\ \hline \end{array}$$

25.
$$\begin{array}{r} 3.0018 \\ 2.9257 \\ 4.63 \\ + 5.0578 \\ \hline \end{array}$$

23. _____

24. _____

25. _____

Name   Score

Solve.

1.   You pay $819.12 for car insurance,   2.   Through a clothing catalogue, you   1. _____
     $1258.75 for health insurance, and   purchased a bathrobe for $24.65, a pair of
     $617.20 for house insurance annually.   slippers for $7.98, and a shirt for $19.95.
     Find the total amount spent annually on   Find the total bill for the clothing.
     insurance.
                                                                                                  2. _____

3.   Find the length of the shaft.   4.   It snowed for three consecutive days. It   3. _____
     1.59 feet   2.66 feet   snowed 1.4 feet the first day, 0.3 feet the
                                                       second day, and 2.25 feet the third day.
           3.2 feet   Find the total snowfall for the three days.

              Length   4. _____

5.   An athlete bicycle 17.2 miles on Monday,   6.   The odometer of your car read 2456.2   5. _____
     6.7 miles on Tuesday, and 12.4 miles on   miles. You drive 65.4 miles on Friday,
     Wednesday. What was the total distance   56.9 miles on Saturday, and 73.3 miles on
     traveled for the three days?   Sunday. Find your odometer reading at the
                                                       end of the three days.
                                                                                                  6. _____

7.   You have $3641.59 in your checking   8.   You have $821.65 in your checking   7. _____
     account. You make deposits of $156.43,   account. You make deposits of $671.46,
     $341.97, $23.21, and $642.76. Find the $88.90, $46.63, and $261.27. Find the
     amount in your checking account after   amount in your checking account after
     making the deposits.   making the deposits.
                                                                                                  8. _____

9.   The deductions from a lab technician's   10. A sales person's commission checks   9. _____
     weekly paycheck are as follows: $92.76 for   for six months are: $3259.04, $5462.36,
     taxes, $6.34 for insurance, and $21.25 for $3423.96, $1350.98, $4812.74, and
     the company savings plan. Find the total $3972.12. Find the total commission
     weekly deduction.   income for the six months.
                                                                                                  10. _____

Name   Score

Subtract and check.

1. $46.287 - 13.91$

2. $23.031 - 17.61$

3. $145.03 - 8.2174$

4. $650 - 56.413$

5. $14.1 - 11.7809$

6. $43.001 - 19.875$

7. $143.24 - 80.794$

8. $9.08 - 6.324$

9. $16.8263 - 9.93$

10.
$$\begin{array}{r} 0.452 \\ -\ 0.39 \\ \hline \end{array}$$

11.
$$\begin{array}{r} 0.847 \\ -\ 0.25 \\ \hline \end{array}$$

12.
$$\begin{array}{r} 9.406 \\ -\ 6.315 \\ \hline \end{array}$$

13.
$$\begin{array}{r} 28.72 \\ -\ 6.318 \\ \hline \end{array}$$

14.
$$\begin{array}{r} 0.17 \\ -\ 0.0093 \\ \hline \end{array}$$

15.
$$\begin{array}{r} 5.002 \\ -\ 3.194 \\ \hline \end{array}$$

16.
$$\begin{array}{r} 177.31 \\ -\ 42.126 \\ \hline \end{array}$$

17.
$$\begin{array}{r} 641 \\ -\ 279.312 \\ \hline \end{array}$$

18.
$$\begin{array}{r} 378.2 \\ -\ 29.458 \\ \hline \end{array}$$

19.
$$\begin{array}{r} 45.701 \\ -\ 8.6225 \\ \hline \end{array}$$

20.
$$\begin{array}{r} 31.006 \\ -\ 12.7196 \\ \hline \end{array}$$

21.
$$\begin{array}{r} 256.87 \\ -\ 75.684 \\ \hline \end{array}$$

22.
$$\begin{array}{r} 441.373 \\ -\ 48.1356 \\ \hline \end{array}$$

23.
$$\begin{array}{r} 729.338 \\ -\ 95.8976 \\ \hline \end{array}$$

24.
$$\begin{array}{r} 32 \\ -\ 27.9841 \\ \hline \end{array}$$

25.
$$\begin{array}{r} 94.05621 \\ -\ 59.30712 \\ \hline \end{array}$$

26.
$$\begin{array}{r} 7.65039 \\ -\ 1.04882 \\ \hline \end{array}$$

27.
$$\begin{array}{r} 83.66215 \\ -\ 41.59876 \\ \hline \end{array}$$

1. _____
2. _____
3. _____
4. _____
5. _____
6. _____
7. _____
8. _____
9. _____
10. _____
11. _____
12. _____
13. _____
14. _____
15. _____
16. _____
17. _____
18. _____
19. _____
20. _____
21. _____
22. _____
23. _____
24. _____
25. _____
26. _____
27. _____

Name _____   Score _____

Solve.

1. You buy a toaster for $16.83. How much change do you receive from a $20.00 bill?

2. A plane takes 0.021 inch off a board that is 1.6 inches thick. Find the resulting thickness of the board.

1. _____

2. _____

3. You bought a 5.3-pound roast. After you trimmed the fat, 3.5 pounds of meat remained. How much fat did you trim from the roast?

4. A competitive swimmer beat the team's record time of 56.27 seconds in the 100-meter freestyle competition by 0.89 seconds. What is the new record time?

3. _____

4. _____

5. During an experiment, a chemist noted that the temperature of a solution rose 5.75° the first minute and then rose another 7.5° the second minute. If the temperature of the solution was 38.25° after the first two minutes, what was the original temperature of the solution?

6. You had a balance of $895.60 in your checking account. You then wrote checks for $45.89, $5.79, and $19.50. Find the new balance in the checking account.

5. _____

6. _____

7. You had a balance of $1263.49 in your checking account. You then wrote checks for $54.91, $27.55, and $283.76. Find the new balance in the checking account.

8. You buy groceries for $32.78, shoes for $25.80, and a shirt for $16.95. How much change do you have left from a $100 bill?

7. _____

8. _____

9. A neighborhood deli had a monthly income of $7320.98 and expenses of $4600.29. Find the profit for the month.

10. A tax accountant has an income of $43,796.52 and pays $9,248.73 in taxes. Find the after tax income.

9. _____

10. _____

Name   Score

Multiply.

1.   0.5   **2.**   6.4   **3.**   5.6   **1.** _____
       × 0.7   × 0.3   ×   9
                                                                                  2. _____

                                                                                  3. _____

4.   0.57   **5.**   0.28   **6.**   5.1   **4.** _____
       ×   4   × 0.6   × 4.5
                                                                                  5. _____

                                                                                  6. _____

7.   0.96   **8.**   2.63   **9.**   5.83   **7.** _____
       × 3.7   × 0.03   × 0.008
                                                                                  8. _____

                                                                                  9. _____

10.   0.67   **11.**   52.9   **12.**   1.07   **10.** _____
       × 0.41   × 0.2   × 0.066
                                                                                 11. _____

                                                                                 12. _____

13.   24.8   **14.**   7.673   **15.**   0.314   **13.** _____
       × 0.0019   × 0.45   × 0.061
                                                                                 14. _____

                                                                                 15. _____

16. 5.92×0.8 **17.** 0.76×0.6 **18.** 3.9×0.44 **16.** _____

                                                                                 17. _____

                                                                                 18. _____

19. 8.21×10 **20.** 0.035×100 **21.** 6.8235×1000 **19.** _____

                                                                                 20. _____

                                                                                 21. _____

22. 6.85×10^1 **23.** 0.035×10^2 **24.** 3.4×10^4 **22.** _____

                                                                                 23. _____

                                                                                 24. _____

25.   3.278   **26.**   2.073   **27.**   0.063   **25.** _____
       ×   4.6   ×   9.5   × 0.34
                                                                                 26. _____

                                                                                 27. _____

Name _____ Score _____

Solve. Round to the nearest cent.

1. A sheet of plywood is 0.25 inch thick. Find the height of a stack of 150 sheets of plywood.

2. A shuttle bus transports students from a suburban college to work study jobs in the city and back again 5 times a day. If the distance between the college and the city is 11.3 miles, find the distance the shuttle bus travels in one day.

1. _____

2. _____

3. The cost of operating an electric saw for one hour is $0.062. How much does it cost to operate the motor for 55 hours?

4. Some states charge a meal tax on the food sold by restaurants. The tax in one state is found my multiplying the cost of the meal by 0.05. The mean you order at a restaurant costs $12.95. Find the total cost of the meal and tax.

3. _____

4. _____

5. A car is bought for $3600 down and payments of $141.50 each month for 24 months. Find the total cost of the car.

6. An inventory clerk earns a salary of $408 for a 40-hour work week. This week the clerk worked 7 hours of overtime at a rate of $15.30 for each hour of overtime. Find the inventory clerk's total income for this week.

5. _____

6. _____

7. You obtain a simple interest loan of $2450. The interest on the loan after one year is found my multiplying the loan amount by 0.12. Find the total amount due at the end of one year.

8. A nurse earns $811.20 for a 40-hour work week. This week the nurse worked 6 hours of overtime at a rate of $25.70 for each hour of overtime worked. Find the nurse's total income for the week.

7. _____

8. _____

9. You bought a house with payments of $1534.25 per month for 25 years. Find the total amount of the payments.

10. You bought a house with payments of $1024.50 per month for 20 years. Find the amount of the payments.

9. _____

10. _____

Name _____   Score _____

Divide.

1. $6\overline{)5.64}$ 2. $0.7\overline{)2.24}$ 3. $0.8\overline{)40}$

4. $0.3\overline{)25.95}$ 5. $5\overline{)6.515}$ 6. $2.9\overline{)0.899}$

7. $0.46\overline{)1.288}$ 8. $0.09\overline{)42.3}$ 9. $0.012\overline{)0.1116}$

Divide. Round to the nearest tenth.

10. $73.85 \div 9.6$ 11. $0.473 \div 0.54$ 12. $1.265 \div 0.043$

Divide. Round to the nearest hundredth.

13. $4.724 \div 17$ 14. $8 \div 0.41$ 15. $36.597 \div 53.2$

Divide. Round to the nearest thousandth.

16. $0.0717 \div 0.9$ 17. $69.418 \div 83.5$ 18. $0.4728 \div 57.5$

Divide. Round to the nearest whole number.

19. $34.19 \div 36$ 20. $6.25 \div 0.4$ 21. $5.125 \div 0.073$

Divide.

22. $7.23 \div 10$ 23. $49.875 \div 10^2$ 24. $3.7615 \div 10^3$

25. $53.072 \div 2.14$ 26. $2.898 \div 0.92$ 27. $0.01878 \div 0.03$

1. _____
2. _____
3. _____
4. _____
5. _____
6. _____
7. _____
8. _____
9. _____
10. _____
11. _____
12. _____
13. _____
14. _____
15. _____
16. _____
17. _____
18. _____
19. _____
20. _____
21. _____
22. _____
23. _____
24. _____
25. _____
26. _____
27. _____

Name   Score

Solve.

1. A file clerk earns $79.20 for working an 8-hour day. How much does the file clerk earn in one hour?

2. An accountant earns $1390.40 for 35.2 hours' work. How much does the accountant earn in one hour?

1. _____

2. _____

3. You pay $1284.72 per year in life insurance premiums. You pay the premiums in 12 equal monthly payments. Find the amount of each monthly payment.

4. Gasoline tax is $0.19 per gallon. Find the number of gallons used during a month in which $518.84 was paid in taxes.

3. _____

4. _____

5. A tax of $1.39 is paid on each hair dryer sold by a store. This month the total tax paid on hair dryers was $31.97. How many hair dryers were sold?

6. A jogger ran 6.8 miles in 42.16 minutes. What was the jogger's average time per mile?

5. _____

6. _____

7. A $7,815.04 car can be bought for a down payment of $2677 and 36 equal monthly payments. Find the amount of each monthly payment.

8. Under the terms of your school loan, you must pay back a total of $15,655.20 over a ten-year period. What are your monthly payments?

7. _____

8. _____

9. A software company has 2,500,00 shares of stock. The company paid $8,125,000 in dividends. Find the dividend for each share of stock.

10. A 15.5-foot board is cut into pieces 3.3 feet long for a bookcase. What is the length of the piece remaining after cutting as many shelves as possible?

9. _____

10. _____

Name   Score

Convert the fraction to a decimal. Round to the nearest thousandth.

1. $\dfrac{5}{7}$

2. $\dfrac{1}{15}$

3. $\dfrac{5}{12}$

4. $\dfrac{8}{9}$

5. $\dfrac{3}{14}$

6. $\dfrac{6}{11}$

7. $2\dfrac{10}{17}$

8. $\dfrac{7}{16}$

9. $5\dfrac{2}{3}$

10. $\dfrac{9}{14}$

11. $\dfrac{6}{7}$

12. $\dfrac{5}{4}$

13. $8\dfrac{3}{22}$

14. $15\dfrac{1}{2}$

15. $\dfrac{53}{100}$

16. $\dfrac{35}{8}$

17. $41\dfrac{3}{10}$

18. $1\dfrac{2}{23}$

19. $6\dfrac{1}{3}$

20. $\dfrac{5}{9}$

21. $\dfrac{39}{11}$

22. $27\dfrac{1}{8}$

23. $\dfrac{46}{7}$

24. $\dfrac{13}{1000}$

25. $\dfrac{17}{18}$

26. $6\dfrac{5}{9}$

27. $10\dfrac{12}{21}$

1. _____
2. _____
3. _____
4. _____
5. _____
6. _____
7. _____
8. _____
9. _____
10. _____
11. _____
12. _____
13. _____
14. _____
15. _____
16. _____
17. _____
18. _____
19. _____
20. _____
21. _____
22. _____
23. _____
24. _____
25. _____
26. _____
27. _____

Name _____   Score _____

Convert the decimal to a fraction.

1. 0.7   **2.** 0.5   **3.** 0.46

4. 0.74   **5.** 0.375   **6.** 0.205

7. 2.55   **8.** 6.75   **9.** 18.4

10. 12.3   **11.** 9.2   **12.** 14.5

13. 4.138   **14.** 6.064   **15.** 3.35

16. 9.93   **17.** $0.16\frac{4}{7}$ **18.** $0.93\frac{1}{3}$

19. $0.11\frac{1}{9}$ **20.** 4.81   **21.** 0.055

22. 0.015   **23.** 23.62   **24.** 0.44

25. $0.83\frac{1}{3}$ **26.** $0.25\frac{1}{6}$ **27.** $0.77\frac{7}{9}$

1. _____
2. _____
3. _____
4. _____
5. _____
6. _____
7. _____
8. _____
9. _____
10. _____
11. _____
12. _____
13. _____
14. _____
15. _____
16. _____
17. _____
18. _____
19. _____
20. _____
21. _____
22. _____
23. _____
24. _____
25. _____
26. _____
27. _____

Name   Score

Place the correct symbol, < or >, between the numbers.

1.   0.23   0.3   2.   0.45   0.5   3.   4.54   4.45

4.   7.10   7.01   5.   9.143   9.134   6.   0.091   0.101

7.   0.399 $\dfrac{2}{5}$ 8.   0.433 $\dfrac{7}{16}$ 9. $\dfrac{5}{9}$ 0.54

10.   0.58 $\dfrac{7}{12}$ 11. $\dfrac{5}{7}$ 0.72   12.   0.26 $\dfrac{4}{15}$

13. $\dfrac{1}{3}$ 0.32   14. $\dfrac{13}{16}$ 0.82   15.   0.626 $\dfrac{5}{8}$

16.   0.4103   0.413   17.   0.25   0.256   18.   0.63   0.063

19.   0.3   1.003   20.   0.7   0.079   21.   0.86   0.859

22. $\dfrac{1}{8}$ 0.124   23. $\dfrac{11}{15}$ 0.734   24.   0.589 $\dfrac{3}{5}$

25.   0.708 $\dfrac{17}{24}$ 26.   0.167 $\dfrac{1}{6}$ 27. $\dfrac{4}{7}$ 0.572

1. _____
2. _____
3. _____
4. _____
5. _____
6. _____
7. _____
8. _____
9. _____
10. _____
11. _____
12. _____
13. _____
14. _____
15. _____
16. _____
17. _____
18. _____
19. _____
20. _____
21. _____
22. _____
23. _____
24. _____
25. _____
26. _____
27. _____

Name

Score

Write the comparison as a ratio in simplest form using a fraction, a colon (:), and the word *to*.

1.	3 yards to 7 yards	2.	6 minutes to 16 minutes	1.	_____
				2.	_____
3.	12 months to 20 months	4.	33 tons to 44 tons	3.	_____
				4.	_____
5.	3 cents to 21 cents	6.	15 inches to 35 inches	5.	_____
				6.	_____
7.	20 days to 4 days	8.	23 quarts to 14 quarts	7.	_____
				8.	_____
9.	5 feet to 5 feet	10.	9 hours to 6 hours	9.	_____
				10.	_____
11.	$7 to $4	12.	12 pints to 36 pints	11.	_____
				12.	_____
13.	60 ounces to 55 ounces	14.	2 cups to 10 cups	13.	_____
				14.	_____
15.	28 pounds to 32 pounds	16.	70 years to 63 years	15.	_____
				16.	_____
17.	9 tons to 12 tons	18.	5 ounces to 11 ounces	17.	_____
				18.	_____
19.	14 days to 12 days	20.	3 minutes to 18 minutes	19.	_____
				20.	_____
21.	43 years to 86 years	22.	32 hours to 20 hours	21.	_____
				22.	_____
23.	27 feet to 12 feet	24.	$16 to $16	23.	_____
				24.	_____
25.	9 pounds to 10 pounds	26.	60 cents to 24 cents	25.	_____
				26.	_____

57

Name   Score

Solve.

1. You sleep 6 hours per day. Find the
    ratio of the number of hours you sleep to
    the number of hours in one day.

2. A bank cashed 176 checks on Thursday
    and 256 checks on Friday. Find the ratio
    of the number of checks cashed on
    Thursday to the number cashed on
    Friday.

1. _____

2. _____

3. In Rhode Island, the average summer and
    winter temperatures are 72°F and 28°F,
    respectively. Find the ratio of the summer
    temperature to the winter temperature.

4. For one month, a family spent $320 for
    food, and $720 for rent. Find the ratio of
    the amount spent for food to the amount
    spent for rent.

3. _____

4. _____

5. During one month, a furniture store sold
    240 bedroom sets and 144 dining room
    sets. Find the ratio of dining room sets
    sold to the number of bedroom sets sold.

6. A home computer that sold for $2400 two
    years ago is now selling for $900. What is
    the ratio of the decrease in price to the
    original price?

5. _____

6. _____

7. Children in a town sold charity raffle
    tickets on Friday and Saturday. They sold
    151 tickets on Friday and 453 tickets on
    Saturday. What is the ratio of the number
    of tickets sold on Saturday to the total
    number of tickets sold on both days?

8. A new homeowner bought a dining room
    table for $336 and 6 chairs for $92 each.
    What is the ratio for the total cost of the 6
    chairs to the total cost of the dining room
    set?

7. _____

8. _____

9. The original value for a compact car was
    $7250. Two years later the car had a value
    of $5750. What is the ratio of the decrease
    in value to the original value?

10. A house had an original value of $72,000
    but increased in value to $93,600 two years
    later. What is the ratio of the increase in
    value to the original value?

9. _____

10. _____

Name _____ Score _____

Write as a rate in simplest form.

1.   106 miles in 4 hours

2.   182 miles on 6 gallons of gasoline

3.   78 feet in 9 seconds

4. $310 for 15 toasters

5. $606 earned in 40 hours

6. $78 for 26 pounds

7. $2004 for 100 shares of stock

8.   4 tablets in 24 hours

9.   726 words in 12 minutes

10. $9150 earned in 6 months

11.   343 miles in 7 hours

12.   5512 words on 24 pages

13. $117 for 18 boards

14.   675 clams for 225 people

15. $10,816 earned in 26 weeks

16.   272 place settings on 34 tables

17.   615 pounds on 45 square inches

18. $203 for 29 feet

19. $5824 distributed among 4 departments

20.   868 seats in 8 lecture halls

21.   2144 miles on 64 gallons of gasoline

22.   570 calls in 12 hours

23.   135 cups of coffee in 9 urns

24.   156 houses on 612 acres

25.   1589 words on 14 pages

26. $247 for 19 pounds

1. _____
2. _____
3. _____
4. _____
5. _____
6. _____
7. _____
8. _____
9. _____
10. _____
11. _____
12. _____
13. _____
14. _____
15. _____
16. _____
17. _____
18. _____
19. _____
20. _____
21. _____
22. _____
23. _____
24. _____
25. _____
26. _____

Name _____   Score _____

Write as a unit rate.

1. $30 for 12 feet   2.   323 miles on 7 gallons   1. _____

                                                                               2. _____

3.   402 pounds on 24 square inches   4. $72,000 for 3 partners   3. _____

                                                                               4. _____

5.   126 gallons in 15 minutes   6.   498 miles in 10 hours   5. _____

                                                                               6. _____

7.   558 feet in 25 seconds   8. $36 for 40 lbs   7. _____

                                                                               8. _____

9.   620 miles in 4 days   10. 204 heartbeats in 3 minutes   9. _____

                                                                               10. _____

11. $18,000 earned in 12 months   12. 352 words in 5.5 minutes   11. _____

                                                                               12. _____

13. $360.96 earned in 35.25 hours   14. $15.52 for 16 plants   13. _____

                                                                               14. _____

15. 455.01 miles in 8.7 hours   16. 536.55 pounds on 73.5 square inches 15. _____

                                                                               16. _____

17. $87.87 for 25.25 pounds   18. 216 words in 4.5 minutes   17. _____

                                                                               18. _____

19. 980.4 gallons in 17.2 minutes   20. 318.6 miles in 10.8 gallons   19. _____

                                                                               20. _____

21. $500 for 4 partners   22. $166.32 earned in 24.75 hours   21. _____

                                                                               22. _____

23. 252 heartbeats in 3.5 minutes   24. 888.3 miles in 7 days   23. _____

                                                                               24. _____

25. $9000 earned in 8 months   26. 1107 feet in 90 seconds   25. _____

                                                                               26. _____

Name _____   Score _____

Solve. Round to the nearest hundredth.

1. An actuary makes $1620 in 40 hours. What is the actuary's wage per hour?

2. Twenty-four feet of lumber cost $62.16. What is the cost per foot?

1. _____

2. _____

3. During a city-wide power outage, the police station logged 651 calls in 5.25 hours. How many calls did the police station receive per hour?

4. A secretary typed a letter with 342 words in 6 minutes. Find the number of words typed in 1 minute.

3. _____

4. _____

5. A grocery store sells 3 pounds of grapes for $2.00. What is the cost of 1 pound?

6. During a sale, the house wares department of a store sold 48 coffee mugs for a total of $95.04. Find the cost per mug.

5. _____

6. _____

7. An investor purchased 350 shares of stock for $29,250. What is the cost per share?

8. A store bought 175 dish towels wholesale for $152.25 and sold them for $243.25. What was the store's profit per towel?

7. _____

8. _____

9. A company with 1,340,000 shares of stock distributed $2,412,000 in dividends. Find the dividend per share.

10. The total cost of making 5000 CDs was $6027. Of the CDs made, 100 did not meet company standards. What was the cost per CD for those CDs which met company standards?

9. _____

10. _____

Name   Score

Determine if the proportion is true or not true.

1. $\dfrac{6}{7} = \dfrac{12}{14}$

2. $\dfrac{15}{9} = \dfrac{25}{15}$

3. $\dfrac{9}{18} = \dfrac{12}{24}$

4. $\dfrac{16}{5} = \dfrac{80}{35}$

5. $\dfrac{3}{30} = \dfrac{11}{110}$

6. $\dfrac{25}{4} = \dfrac{80}{14}$

7. $\dfrac{6}{8} = \dfrac{34}{46}$

8. $\dfrac{8}{2} = \dfrac{36}{9}$

9. $\dfrac{4}{5} = \dfrac{15}{16}$

10. $\dfrac{7}{10} = \dfrac{35}{50}$

11. $\dfrac{24}{33} = \dfrac{34}{44}$

12. $\dfrac{18}{10} = \dfrac{63}{34}$

13. $\dfrac{133 \text{ miles}}{3 \text{ hours}} = \dfrac{622 \text{ miles}}{14 \text{ hours}}$

14. $\dfrac{21 \text{ feet}}{5 \text{ seconds}} = \dfrac{63 \text{ feet}}{15 \text{ seconds}}$

15. $\dfrac{606 \text{ words}}{10 \text{ minutes}} = \dfrac{302 \text{ words}}{5 \text{ minutes}}$

16. $\dfrac{48 \text{ cents}}{4 \text{ hours}} = \dfrac{60 \text{ cents}}{5 \text{ hours}}$

17. $\dfrac{238 \text{ miles}}{7 \text{ gallons}} = \dfrac{476 \text{ miles}}{12 \text{ gallons}}$

18. $\dfrac{\$600}{36 \text{ hours}} = \dfrac{\$400}{24 \text{ hours}}$

19. $\dfrac{155 \text{ minutes}}{25 \text{ miles}} = \dfrac{341 \text{ minutes}}{55 \text{ miles}}$

20. $\dfrac{126 \text{ calls}}{6 \text{ hours}} = \dfrac{86 \text{ calls}}{4 \text{ hours}}$

21. $\dfrac{282 \text{ houses}}{47 \text{ acres}} = \dfrac{188 \text{ houses}}{33 \text{ acres}}$

22. $\dfrac{450 \text{ gallons}}{60 \text{ minutes}} = \dfrac{180 \text{ gallons}}{24 \text{ minutes}}$

23. $\dfrac{6200 \text{ words}}{40 \text{ pages}} = \dfrac{7750 \text{ words}}{50 \text{ pages}}$

24. $\dfrac{375 \text{ cars}}{250 \text{ people}} = \dfrac{1218 \text{ cars}}{312 \text{ people}}$

25. $\dfrac{\$17{,}520}{12 \text{ months}} = \dfrac{\$43{,}800}{30 \text{ months}}$

26. $\dfrac{\$4950}{200 \text{ shares}} = \dfrac{\$6180}{250 \text{ shares}}$

1. _____
2. _____
3. _____
4. _____
5. _____
6. _____
7. _____
8. _____
9. _____
10. _____
11. _____
12. _____
13. _____
14. _____
15. _____
16. _____
17. _____
18. _____
19. _____
20. _____
21. _____
22. _____
23. _____
24. _____
25. _____
26. _____

Name _____   Score _____

Solve. Round to the nearest hundredth.

1. $\dfrac{3}{5} = \dfrac{n}{10}$

2. $\dfrac{n}{8} = \dfrac{20}{32}$

3. $\dfrac{14}{24} = \dfrac{7}{n}$

4. $\dfrac{4}{28} = \dfrac{n}{196}$

5. $\dfrac{21}{n} = \dfrac{14}{16}$

6. $\dfrac{6}{20} = \dfrac{5}{n}$

7. $\dfrac{8}{n} = \dfrac{9}{27}$

8. $\dfrac{13}{36} = \dfrac{39}{n}$

9. $\dfrac{n}{18} = \dfrac{5}{9}$

10. $\dfrac{42}{15} = \dfrac{n}{12}$

11. $\dfrac{n}{8} = \dfrac{9}{12}$

12. $\dfrac{18}{n} = \dfrac{96}{132}$

13. $\dfrac{10}{20} = \dfrac{12}{n}$

14. $\dfrac{5}{11} = \dfrac{n}{9}$

15. $\dfrac{35}{14} = \dfrac{15}{n}$

16. $\dfrac{35}{n} = \dfrac{22}{11}$

17. $\dfrac{90}{n} = \dfrac{36}{3}$

18. $\dfrac{8}{18} = \dfrac{2}{n}$

19. $\dfrac{19}{n} = \dfrac{54}{135}$

20. $\dfrac{n}{28} = \dfrac{42}{18}$

21. $\dfrac{30}{n} = \dfrac{24}{14}$

22. $\dfrac{n}{15} = \dfrac{0.8}{5.6}$

23. $\dfrac{1.8}{18} = \dfrac{n}{12}$

24. $\dfrac{3.4}{20} = \dfrac{5.1}{n}$

25. $\dfrac{13.9}{n} = \dfrac{26.28}{51.7}$

26. $\dfrac{5149}{278} = \dfrac{156}{n}$

27. $\dfrac{n}{4.21} = \dfrac{6.793}{1.248}$

1. _____
2. _____
3. _____
4. _____
5. _____
6. _____
7. _____
8. _____
9. _____
10. _____
11. _____
12. _____
13. _____
14. _____
15. _____
16. _____
17. _____
18. _____
19. _____
20. _____
21. _____
22. _____
23. _____
24. _____
25. _____
26. _____
27. _____

Name _____   Score _____

Solve. Round to the nearest hundredth.

1. A life insurance policy costs $4.52 for every $1000 of insurance. At this rate, what is the cost for $20,000 worth of life insurance?

2. A liquid plant food is prepared by using one gallon of water for each 1.5 teaspoon of plant food. At this rate, how many teaspoons of plant food are required for 7 gallons of water?

1. _____

2. _____

3. A $19.75 sales tax is charged for a $395 purchase. At this rate, what is the sales tax for a $621 purchase?

4. The scale on the plans for a new office building is 1 inch equals 4 feet. How long is a room that measures $8\frac{1}{2}$ inches on the drawing?

3. _____

4. _____

5. A stock investment of 150 shares paid a dividend of $555. At this rate, what dividend would be paid on 280 shares of stock?

6. A bank demands a loan payment of $18.95 each month for every $1000 borrowed. At this rate, what is the monthly payment for a $6000 loan?

5. _____

6. _____

7. A transistor company expects that 3 out of 245 transistors will be defective. How many defective transistors will be found in a batch of 184,485 transistors?

8. A department store makes a profit of $15.20 on every 25 rolls of film sold. How much profit is made if 16 rolls of film are sold?

7. _____

8. _____

9. For every 10 people who work in a city, 7 of them commute by public transportation. If 34,600 people work in the city, how many of them do not take public transportation?

10. For every 15 gallons of water pumped into the holding tank, 8 gallons were pumped out. After 930 gallons had been pumped in, how much water remained in the tank?

9. _____

10. _____

Name _____ Score _____

Write as a fraction and as a decimal.

1. 39%	**2.** 64%	**3.** 125%	**1.** _____
			2. _____
			3. _____
4. 26%	**5.** 85%	**6.** 20%	**4.** _____
			5. _____
			6. _____
7. 450%	**8.** 19%	**9.** 55%	**7.** _____
			8. _____
			9. _____

Write as a fraction.

10. $7\frac{8}{9}\%$	**11.** $7\frac{2}{3}\%$	**12.** $25\frac{4}{5}\%$	**10.** _____
			11. _____
			12. _____
13. $64\frac{1}{2}\%$	**14.** $43\frac{1}{3}\%$	**15.** $99\frac{3}{5}\%$	**13.** _____
			14. _____
			15. _____

Write as a decimal.

16. 67.5%	**17.** 34.07%	**18.** 57.9%	**16.** _____
			17. _____
			18. _____
19. 40%	**20.** 13.89%	**21.** 2.01%	**19.** _____
			20. _____
			21. _____

Name   Score

Write as a percent.

1.   0.32   2.   0.96   3.   0.04   1. _____

                                                                                      2. _____

                                                                                      3. _____

4.   1.97   5.   2.14   6.   0.009   4. _____

                                                                                      5. _____

                                                                                      6. _____

7.   0.68   8.   0.12   9.   0.107   7. _____

                                                                                      8. _____

                                                                                      9. _____

Write as a percent. Round to the nearest tenth.

10. $\dfrac{25}{60}$ 11. $1\dfrac{8}{9}$ 12. $\dfrac{4}{7}$ 10. _____

                                                                                      11. _____

                                                                                      12. _____

13. $64\dfrac{1}{2}\%$ 14. $\dfrac{3}{5}$ 15. $1\dfrac{5}{6}$ 13. _____

                                                                                      14. _____

                                                                                      15. _____

Write as a percent. Write the remainder in fractional form.

16. $\dfrac{5}{11}$ 17. $\dfrac{2}{9}$ 18. $1\dfrac{1}{7}$ 16. _____

                                                                                      17. _____

                                                                                      18. _____

19. $\dfrac{3}{8}$ 20. $\dfrac{1}{15}$ 21. $\dfrac{7}{12}$ 19. _____

                                                                                      20. _____

                                                                                      21. _____

Name   Score

Solve.

1. 8% of 45 is what?   2. 15% of 100 is what?   1. _____

                                                                 2. _____

3. 26% of 70 is what?   4. 53% of 90 is what?   3. _____

                                                                 4. _____

5. What is 45% of 60?   6. What is 35% of 55?   5. _____

                                                                 6. _____

7. What is 65% of 135.5?   8. What is 52% of 24.4?   7. _____

                                                                 8. _____

9. What is 4% of 2800?   10. What is 0.02% of 250?   9. _____

                                                                 10. _____

11. 5% of 900 is what?   12. 0.025% of 800 is what?   11. _____

                                                                 12. _____

13. 150% of 98 is what?   14. 220% of 6 is what?   13. _____

                                                                 14. _____

15. Find 12% of 540.   16. Find 30% of 17.5.   15. _____

                                                                 16. _____

17. Find 7.9% of 120.   18. Find 2.5% of 440.   17. _____

                                                                 18. _____

19. Find 0.08% of 375   20. Find 25% of 144.   19. _____

                                                                 20. _____

21. What is 12.5% of 1540?   22. What is $6\frac{1}{4}$% of 620?   21. _____

                                                                 22. _____

23. What is $33\frac{1}{3}$% of 591?   24. What is $83\frac{1}{3}$% of 72?   23. _____

                                                                 24. _____

25. 43.18% of 800 is what?   26. 16.83% of 500 is what?   25. _____

                                                                 26. _____

Name   Score

Solve.

1. A company uses 14% of its $55,000 budget for office supplies. What amount of the budget is spent for office supplies?

2. A company survey found that $16\frac{2}{3}\%$ of the employees were dissatisfied with the company's cafeteria. If 2400 employees were surveyed, how many employees were dissatisfied with the cafeteria?

1. _____

2. _____

3. A person purchases a television which costs $259 and pays a sales tax which is 5% of the cost. What is the sales tax on the television?

4. During a power outage, 9% of the city's 46,500 homes were without electricity. How many homes were affected by the power outage?

3. _____

4. _____

5. A nursery sold 450 geranium plants in June. In July, the nursery increased its sales by 8%. How many geranium plants were sold in July?

6. A restaurant serves 35% more ice cream in June than it does in May. How much ice cream does the restaurant serve in June if it serves 12 gallons of ice cream in May?

5. _____

6. _____

7. A quality control inspector found that 0.2% of the 2500 flathead screws inspected were defective. How many screws were not defective?

8. A plumber's hourly wage is $18.50 before an 8% raise. What is the new hourly wage?

7. _____

8. _____

9. A truck retail sales company makes a 5.3% profit on sales of $520,000. Find the profit.

10. An office building has an appraised value of $8,000,000. The real estate taxes are 2.35% of the appraised value of the building. Find the real estate taxes.

9. _____

10. _____

Name _____ Score _____

Solve.

1. What percent of 112 is 35?

2. What percent of 72 is 12?

3. What percent of 75 is 60?

4. What percent of 45 is 27?

5. 17 is what percent of 85?

6. 27 is what percent of 60?

7. What percent of 8 is 24?

8. What percent of 24 is 50?

9. 15 is what percent of 100?

10. 54 is what percent of 150?

11. 135 is what percent of 3000?

12. 48 is what percent of 1200?

13. What percent of 620 is 465?

14. What percent of 130 is 13?

15. What percent of 5 is 1.5?

16. What percent of 3.8 is 0.19?

17. 18.5 is what percent of 3.7?

18. 4.5 is what percent of 40?

19. 0.05 is what percent of 10?

20. 2.444 is what percent of 47?

21. What percent of 9000 is 2745?

22. What percent of 7500 is 2500?

23. 425 is what percent of 2550?

24. 163 is what percent of 815?

25. What percent of 83.2 is 7.904?

26. What percent of 16.85 is 25.275?

1. _____

2. _____

3. _____

4. _____

5. _____

6. _____

7. _____

8. _____

9. _____

10. _____

11. _____

12. _____

13. _____

14. _____

15. _____

16. _____

17. _____

18. _____

19. _____

20. _____

21. _____

22. _____

23. _____

24. _____

25. _____

26. _____

Name _____   Score _____

Solve.

1. A used car salesperson sold 6 of the 50 cars in the lot. What percent of the total number of cars in the lot were sold?

2. An investor received a dividend of $540 on an investment of $4500. What percent of the investment is the dividend?

1. _____

2. _____

3. A company's stock is trading at $55 and pays a dividend of $3.30. What percent of the stock price is the dividend?

4. A home sold for $35,900 in 1972. The same home in 1982 had a value of $82,570. What percent of the 1972 value is the 1982 value?

3. _____

4. _____

5. A survey of 1760 people showed that 352 people favored the incumbent mayor. What percent of the people surveyed favored the incumbent mayor?

6. Of the 3900 resistors tested, 117 were found defective. What percent of the total number of resistors were defective?

5. _____

6. _____

7. A total of $4200 was paid in taxes on an income of $16,800. Find the percent of the total income paid in taxes.

8. An advertising survey of 265 people found that 53 liked a new toothpaste. What percent of the people surveyed did not like the new toothpaste?

7. _____

8. _____

9. A 2.3-acre piece of oceanfront property is appraised at $250,000. The land is bought for $300,000. What percent of the appraised value is the purchase price?

10. A construction company spent $125,000 of its $1,000,000 equipment budget for a bulldozer. What percent of the equipment budget was spent for the bulldozer?

9. _____

10. _____

Name

Score

Solve.

1. 20% of what is 37?

2. 21% of what is 84?

3. 12 is 24% of what?

4. 42 is 70% of what?

5. 12 is 12% of what?

6. 35 is 50% of what?

7. 25% of what is 30.75?

8. 60% of what is 110.4?

9. 3.1% of what is 155?

10. 15.5% of what is 124?

11. 130% of what is 741?

12. 250% of what is 40?

13. 264 is 24% of what?

14. 63 is 18% of what?

15. 1.26 is 2.8% of what?

16. 235.35 is 52.3% of what?

17. 40% of what is 8.4?

18. 68% of what is 136?

19. 0.6% of what is 5.34?

20. 0.75% of what is 12.75?

21. 59 is $66\frac{2}{3}$ % of what?

22. 9.5 is $16\frac{2}{3}$ % of what?

23. 20 is $83\frac{1}{3}$ % of what?

24. 86 is $33\frac{1}{3}$ % of what?

25. 7.5% of what is 4.65?

26. 5.6% of what is 4.382?

1. _____

2. _____

3. _____

4. _____

5. _____

6. _____

7. _____

8. _____

9. _____

10. _____

11. _____

12. _____

13. _____

14. _____

15. _____

16. _____

17. _____

18. _____

19. _____

20. _____

21. _____

22. _____

23. _____

24. _____

25. _____

26. _____

Name   Score

Solve.

1. A used car was purchased for $5750. This was 46% of the new car cost. Find the new car cost.

2. A growing city has 456 business establishments. This is 120% of the number of businesses in the city two years ago. How many business establishments were there in the city two years ago?

3. A student answered 14 of the questions on the two-hour exam incorrectly. This was 25% of the total number of exam questions. How many questions were on the exam?

4. A historian's personal library contains 108 fiction novels. This is 4% of the total number of books in the library. Find the number of books in the historian's library.

5. A police station received 8 calls concerning shoplifting in one day. This was $33\frac{1}{3}$% of the total number of calls received that day. How many calls in all did the police station receive?

6. A carpenter's wage this year is $17.25 an hour. This is 115% of last year's wage. What was the increase in the hourly wage over last year?

7. A company spent $184,000 on advertising in one year. This was 23% of the company's annual budget. What was the company's annual budget?

8. In a parking garage 147 spaces were occupied. This was 98% of the total number of parking spaces. Find the number of unoccupied spaces in the garage.

9. Defects were found in 1659 DVDs. This was 0.21% of the total number of DVDs produced in one month. Find the total number of DVDs produced in that month.

10. An apartment complex is bought for $6,000,000. This is 80% of its appraised value. Find the apartment complex's appraised value.

1. _____

2. _____

3. _____

4. _____

5. _____

6. _____

7. _____

8. _____

9. _____

10. _____

Name   Score

Solve.

1.   34% of 850 is what?   2.   What is 15% of 400?   1. _____

                                                                           2. _____

3.   54 is what percent of 180?   4.   What percent of 120 is 42?   3. _____

                                                                           4. _____

5.   90% of what is 54?   6.   146 is 73% of what?   5. _____

                                                                           6. _____

7.   What percent of 324 is 162?   8.   What percent of 140 is 35?   7. _____

                                                                           8. _____

9.   153 is 30% of what?   10. 7.5% of what is 60?   9. _____

                                                                           10. _____

11. 222 is what percent of 600?   12. 144 is what percent of 32?   11. _____

                                                                           12. _____

13. What is 160% of 480?   14. 210% of 390 is what?   13. _____

                                                                           14. _____

15. 27 is 45% of what?   16. 24% of what is 36?   15. _____

                                                                           16. _____

17. What percent of 110 is 44?   18. 65 is what percent of 125?   17. _____

                                                                           18. _____

19. What percent of 220 is 11?   20. What percent of 72 is 9?   19. _____

                                                                           20. _____

21. 91 is what percent of 26?   22. What percent of 46 is 184?   21. _____

                                                                           22. _____

23. 0.2% of what is 33?   24. 15 is 0.6% of what?   23. _____

                                                                           24. _____

25. Find 1.75% of 8000.   26. 435 is what percent of 6000?   25. _____

                                                                           26. _____

Name   Score

Solve.

1. A soccer team won 51 out of 68 games they played. What percent of the games played did they win?

2. During shipping, 600 of the 4800 light bulbs were damaged. What percent of the number of light bulbs were damaged in the shipping?

3. A supermarket reduced the price of roast beef to $2.24 per pound, which is 80% of the original price. What was the original price?

4. A growing company reinvested 63% of the $120,000 it earned into research and development. How much of the money earned was reinvested into research and development?

5. A monthly state income tax is 12% of the amount earned over $1800. What state income tax does a person pay on a salary of $3000?

6. During an inspection of 120 motorcycles, 3 of them did not pass the safety test. What percent of the motorcycles inspected did pass the safety test?

7. A down payment of $1305 was paid on a new car. The down payment is 15% of the cost of the car. Find the cost of the car.

8. An administrative assistant types 70 words per minute with 98% accuracy. During 5 minutes of typing, how many errors does the secretary make?

9. You bought a boat one year ago. Since then it has depreciated to $1018.50, which is 9.7% of the price you paid for it. How much did you pay for the boat?

10. A down payment of $15,600 was paid on a new house costing $78,000. What percent of the purchase price is the down payment?

1. _____

2. _____

3. _____

4. _____

5. _____

6. _____

7. _____

8. _____

9. _____

10. _____

Name   Score

Find the unit cost. Round to the nearest tenth of a cent.

1. Salad dressing,
    8 ounces for $1.16

2. Non-dairy creamer,
    11 ounces for $1.42

3. Soup,
    $10\frac{1}{2}$ ounces for $0.36

4. Grape juice,
    64 ounces for $1.78

5. Black pepper,
    2 ounces for $0.63

6. Peanut butter,
    28 ounces for $2.62

7. Bouillon cubes,
    15 for $0.59

8. Shampoo,
    15 ounces for $2.87

9. Detergent,
    49 ounces for $1.79

10. Crackers,
    7 ounces for $1.13

11. Anti-freeze,
    64 ounces for $4.99

12. Fried chicken,
    15 pieces for $8.99

13. Pot pies,
    3 for $0.89

14. Corn chips,
    7 ounces for $1.39

15. Bagels,
    8 for $0.79

16. Shoe polish,
    $3\frac{1}{2}$ ounces for $1.48

17. Spaghetti,
    16 ounces for $0.54

18. Potatoes,
    5 pounds for $1.29

19. Spray starch,
    22 ounces for $1.29

20. Clothes pins,
    24 for $1.29

21. Bread,
    16 ounces for $0.88

22. Photograph processing,
    24 pictures for $10.08

23. Cat food,
    18 ounces for $0.94

24. Shortening,
    3 pounds for $2.69

1. _____
2. _____
3. _____
4. _____
5. _____
6. _____
7. _____
8. _____
9. _____
10. _____
11. _____
12. _____
13. _____
14. _____
15. _____
16. _____
17. _____
18. _____
19. _____
20. _____
21. _____
22. _____
23. _____
24. _____

Name   Score

Find the more economical purchase.

1. Syrup,
   15 ounces for $0.94 or
   24 ounces for $1.51

2. Grape jelly,
   32 ounces for $1.29 or
   24 ounces for $0.94

3. Franks,
   16 ounces for $1.79 or
   12 ounces for $1.30

4. Facial tissue,
   175 for $0.79 or
   125 for $0.63

5. Aspirins,
   50 for $1.89 or
   75 for $3.00

6. Yogurt,
   6 ounces for $0.46 or
   10 ounces for $0.74

7. Cream cheese,
   8 ounces for $0.89 or
   12 ounces for $1.39

8. Peanut butter,
   18 ounces for $1.39 or
   22 ounces for $1.75

9. Orange juice,
   64 ounces for $1.35 or
   12 ounces for $0.33

10. Light bulbs,
    4 for $1.99 or
    6 for $3.11

11. Razor blades,
    9 for $1.27 or
    12 for $1.74

12. Ice cream,
    32 ounces for $2.79 or
    16 ounces for $1.44

13. Coffee,
    16 ounces for $2.49 or
    12 ounces for $2.16

14. Flour,
    5 pounds for $0.89 or
    2 pounds for $0.35

15. Mushrooms,
    8 ounces for $0.99 or
    2.5 ounces for $0.35

16. Charcoal,
    10 pounds for $2.67 or
    5 pounds for $1.35

17. Bread,
    24 ounces for $0.93 or
    18 ounces for $0.54

18. Frozen lemonade,
    6 ounces for $0.39 or
    12 ounces for $0.79

19. Sandwich bags,
    50 bags for $1.09 or
    60 bags for $1.44

20. Liquid detergent,
    9 ounces for $0.69 or
    6.5 ounces for $0.39

21. Biscuits,
    9 ounces for $0.59 or
    14 ounces for $0.92

22. Paper towels,
    119 sheets for $0.79 or
    144 sheets for $0.96

23. Cheese slices,
    12 ounces for $1.27 or
    8 ounces for $0.89

24. Bacon,
    12 ounces for $1.28 or
    20 ounces for $2.19

1. _____

2. _____

3. _____

4. _____

5. _____

6. _____

7. _____

8. _____

9. _____

10. _____

11. _____

12. _____

13. _____

14. _____

15. _____

16. _____

17. _____

18. _____

19. _____

20. _____

21. _____

22. _____

23. _____

24. _____

Name   Score

Solve.

1. Pork chops cost $1.79 per pound. Find the cost of 4 pounds.

2. Decorative stepping stones cost $1.15 per stone. Find the cost of 24 stones.

3. Honeydew melons cost $1.99 each. Find the total cost of 4 melons.

4. Grapes cost $0.68 per pound. Find The cost of 2.8 pounds. Round to the nearest cent.

5. Potato chips cost 12.3¢ per ounce. Find the cost of 9.5 ounces. Round to the nearest cent.

6. Salami costs $3.49 per pound. Find the cost of 0.85 pounds. Round to the nearest cent.

7. Carrots cost $0.41 per pound. Find The total cost of 1.6 pounds. Round to the nearest cent.

8. Baked ham costs $3.59 per pound. Find the total cost of 3.2 pounds. Round to the nearest cent.

9. Peanuts cost $2.00 per pound. Find the total cost of $\frac{5}{8}$ pounds.

10. Motor oil costs $1.18 per quart. Find the cost of 6 quarts of oil.

11. A two-piece meal of fried chicken costs $2.65. Find the total cost of 4 two-piece meals.

12. Raisins cost $1.79 per pound. Find the total cost of 0.75 pounds. Round to the nearest cent.

13. Heavy duty lawn bags cost $2.49 per package. How much change do you receive from $20.00 when purchasing 4 packages of lawn bags?

14. Plywood costs $9.99 per sheet. How much change do you receive from $50.00 when purchasing 4 sheets of plywood?

15. Redwood stains costs $12.50 per gallon. How much change do you receive from $50.00 when purchasing 3 gallons?

16. Top soil costs $37.50 per truck load. How much change do you receive from $100.00 when purchasing 2 truck loads of top soil?

1. _____

2. _____

3. _____

4. _____

5. _____

6. _____

7. _____

8. _____

9. _____

10. _____

11. _____

12. _____

13. _____

14. _____

15. _____

16. _____

Name _____   Score _____

Solve. Round to the nearest tenth of a percent or to the nearest tenth of a cent.

1. The value of a $7000 investment increased $1750. What percent increase does this represent?

2. A sweater which sold for $24 last month increased in price by $2. What percent increase does this represent?

1. _____

2. _____

3. The average price of fuel oil rose from $0.75 to $1.00 in six months. What was the percent increase in the price of fuel oil?

4. The number of students enrolled in a speed reading course increased from 60 to 66 during the first 10 days of school. What is the percent increase?

3. _____

4. _____

5. A manufacturer of ceiling fans increased its monthly out put of 1500 by 10%. What is the amount of increase?

6. An advertising agency increased its 200 billboards by 15% during the past year. How many billboards does the agency have now?

5. _____

6. _____

7. The employees of a manufacturing plant received a 6% increase in pay.
    a. What is the amount of the increase for an employee who makes $225 per week?
    b. What is the weekly wage for the employee after the wage increase?

8. A supervisor's salary this year is $32,000. This salary will increase by 8% next year.
    a. What is the amount of increase?
    b. What will the salary be next year?

7. a. _____

b. _____

8. a. _____

b. _____

9. A college increased its number of parking spaces from 1000 to 1050.
    a. How many new spaces were added?
    b. What percent increase does this represent?

10. A town plans to increase its 4000 water meters by 7.5%.
    a. How many more water meters is this?
    b. What will the total number of water meters be after this increase?

9. a. _____

b. _____

10. a. _____

b. _____

11. A cafeteria increased the number of items on the menu from 80 to 90. What percent of increase does this represent?

12. The amount of gasoline used by a fleet of cars increased from 200 to 230 gallons per day. What percent increase does this represent?

11. _____

12. _____

Name _____   Score _____

Solve.

1. A store manager used a markup rate of 30% on all desk lamps. What is the markup on a lamp which costs the store $26?

2. A manager of a natural food store determines that the markup rate of 17% is necessary to make a profit. What is the markup on an item which costs the dealer $2?

1. _____

2. _____

3. An automobile tire dealer uses a markup rate of 32%. What is the markup on tires which cost the dealer $34?

4. The markup on a necklace which costs a jeweler $60 is $36. What markup rate does this represent? (Solve the basic percent equation for percent.)

3. _____

4. _____

5. A beach-wear shop uses a markup rate of 40% on a bathing suit which costs the shop $34.
   a. What is the markup?
   b. What is the selling price?

6. A department store uses a markup rate of 44% on its Model XL food processor which costs the store $45.
   a. What is the markup?
   b. What is the selling price?

5. a. _____

   b. _____

6. a. _____

   b. _____

7. A produce market pays $1.09 for pineapples. The market uses a 55% markup rate.
   a. What is the markup?
   b. What is the selling price?

8. A garden shop uses a markup rate of 35% on a rose trellis which costs the store $26.
   a. What is the markup?
   b. What is the selling price?

7. a. _____

   b. _____

8. a. _____

   b. _____

9. A store uses a markup rate of 38%. What is the selling price for the DVD player which costs the store $47?

10. What is the selling price on a pair of jogging shoes which costs a store $31? The store uses a markup rate of 44%.

9. _____

10. _____

Name _____   Score _____

Solve.

1. A health spa sold 120 memberships in November. In May the spa sold 18 fewer memberships than in November. What was the percent decrease in the number of memberships sold?

2. A new bypass around a small town reduced the normal 40-minute driving time between two cities by 12 minutes. What percent decrease does this represent?

1. _____

2. _____

3. By washing all the clothes in cold water, a family was able to reduce its normal monthly utility bill of $125 by $15. What percent decrease does this represent?

4. By installing solar panels, a copying center reduced its normal $240 per month heating bill by $36. What percent decrease does this represent?

3. _____

4. _____

5. A golf resort employs 180 people during the golfing season. At the end of the season, the resort reduces the number of employees by 45%. What is the decrease in the number of employees?

6. It is estimated that the value of a motorcycle is reduced by 25% after one year of ownership. Using this estimate, how much value does a $1500 new motorcycle lose after one year?

5. _____

6. _____

7. A new process reduced the time needed to replate a piece of silverware from 16 minutes to 10 minutes.
    a. What is the amount of decrease?
    b. What percent decrease does this represent?

8. Because of a decrease in orders for telephones, a telephone center reduced the orders for phones from 140 per month to 91 per month.
    a. What is the amount of decrease?
    b. What percent decrease does this represent?

7. a. _____

   b. _____

8. a. _____

   b. _____

9. Last year a company earned a profit of $285,000. This year, the company's profits were 6% less than last year's.
    a. What was the amount of decrease?
    b. What was the profit this year?

10. Last year, a laptop computer cost $420 to produce. Mass production enabled this manufacturer to reduce this expense by 15%.
    a. What is the amount of decrease?
    b. What percent decrease does this represent?

9. a. _____

   b. _____

10. a. _____

    b. _____

11. The price of a new model digital camera dropped from $150 to $114 in ten months. What percent decrease does this represent?

12. As a result of computerized cash registers, the average customer check-out time has decreased from 10 minutes to 9.5 minutes. What percent decrease does this represent?

11. _____

12. _____

Name _____   Score _____

Solve.

1. To promote business, a store manager offers a small vacuum cleaner which regularly sells for $25 at $9 off the regular price. What is the discount rate?

2. A department store is giving a discount of $6 on an ice chest which normally sells for $40. What is the discount rate?

1. _____

2. _____

3. A sporting goods store is selling its $150 exercise bike for 20% off the regular price. What is the discount?

4. A jewelry store is selling $250 quartz watches at 30% off the regular price. What is the discount?

3. _____

4. _____

5. A stereo speaker set which regularly costs $450 is on sale for $90 off the regular price. What is the discount rate?

6. A hardware store is selling its $32 lock set for 15% off the regular price. What is the discount?

5. _____

6. _____

7. Colby cheese which regularly sells for $2.40 per pound is on sale for 25% off the regular price.
    a. What is the discount?
    b. What is the sale price?

8. The pro shop at the racketball club has its regularly priced $55 shoes on sale for 18% off the regular price.
    a. What is the discount?
    b. What is the sale price?

7. a. _____

   b. _____

8. a. _____

   b. _____

9. A gift shop has its picture frames which regularly cost $35 on sale for $30.80.
    a. What is the discount?
    b. What is the discount rate?

10. An automobile body shop has regularly priced $600 paint jobs on sale for $480.
    a. What is the discount?
    b. What is the discount rate?

9. a. _____

   b. _____

10. a. _____

    b. _____

11. During a going-out-of-business sale, all lawn and garden merchandise was reduced 40% off the regular price. What was the sale price of a lawn mower which normally sells for $230?

12. A store offering 35% off its stock of art supplies. What is the sale price of a set of paint brushes which regularly sells for $60?

11. _____

12. _____

Name   Score

Solve.

1. A rancher borrows $120,000 for 10 months at an annual interest rate of 18%. What is the simple interest due on the loan?

2. To finance the purchase of 8 new taxicabs, the owners of the fleet borrows $84,000 for 8 months at an annual interest rate of 16%. What is the simple interest due on the loan?

3. A mobile home dealer borrowed $160,000 at a 15.5% annual interest rate for four years. What is the simple interest due on the loan?

4. An executive was offered a $34,000 loan at a 14.5% annual interest rate for three years. Find the simple interest due on the loan.

5. You arrange for a 6-month bank loan of $6000 at an annual simple interest rate of 7.5%. Find the total amount you must repay to the bank.

6. A bank charges its customers an interest rate of 1.8% per month for transferring money into an account which is overdrawn. Find the interest owed to the bank for one month when $300 was transferred into an overdrawn account.

7. A copier is purchased and a $2100 loan is obtained for two years at a simple interest rate of 17%.
    a. Find the interest due on the loan.
    b. Find the monthly payment.
    $$\left(\text{Monthly payment} = \frac{\text{loan amount} + \text{interest}}{\text{number of months}}\right)$$

8. An oil well drilling company purchased two new helicopters for $65,000 and financed the full amount at 9% simple annual interest for four years.
    a. Find the interest due on the loan.
    b. Find the monthly payment.
    $$\left(\text{Monthly payment} = \frac{\text{loan amount} + \text{interest}}{\text{number of months}}\right)$$

9. A company purchased a computer system for $75,000 and financed the full amount for five years at a simple annual interest rate of 15%.
    a. Find the interest due on the loan.
    b. Find the monthly payment.

10. To reduce their inventory of new cars, a dealer is offering car loans at a simple annual interest rate of 11%.
    a. Find the interest charged to a customer who financed a car loan of $8200 for four years.
    b. Find the monthly payment.

1. _____

2. _____

3. _____

4. _____

5. _____

6. _____

7. a. _____

   b. _____

8. a. _____

   b. _____

9. a. _____

   b. _____

10. a. _____

    b. _____

Name   Score

Solve.

1. A credit card company charges a customer 1.5% per month on the customer's unpaid balance. Find the interest owed to the credit card company when the customer's unpaid balance for the month is $17,642.59.

2. Suppose you have an unpaid balance of $6753.27 on a credit card that charges 1.25% per month on any unpaid balance. What finance charges do you owe the company?

1. _____

2. _____

3. What is the finance charge on an unpaid balance of $21,453.38 on a credit card that charges 1.75% per month on any unpaid balance?

4. A credit card company charges a customer 1.25% per month on the customer's unpaid balance. Find the interest owed to the credit card company when the customer's unpaid balance for the month is $12,948.71.

3. _____

4. _____

5. Suppose you have an unpaid balance of $9487.43 on a credit card that charges 1.75% per month on any unpaid balance. What finance charges do you owe the company?

6. A credit card customer has an unpaid balance of $1348.56. What is the difference between monthly finance charges of 1.75% per month on the unpaid balance and monthly finance charges of 1.25% per month?

5. _____

6. _____

7. One credit card company charges 1.5% per month on any unpaid balance, and a second company charges 1.25%. What is the difference between the finance charges that these two companies assess on an unpaid balance of $3427.89?

8. You have an unpaid balance of $2675.43. What is the difference between monthly finance charges of 1.5% per month on the unpaid balance and monthly finance charges of 1.75% per month?

7. _____

8. _____

Name   Score

Solve. Use the Compound Interest Table. Round to the nearest cent.

1. An investment of $1750 pays 8%
    annual interest compounded quarterly.
    What is the value of the investment
    after ten years?

2. A time savings deposit pays 15%
    annual interest, compounded daily.
    Find the value of $800 deposited in
    this account after five years.

1. _____

2. _____

3. A money market fund pays 14% annual
    interest, compounded daily. What is
    the value after 15 years of $3000
    invested in this money market fund?

4. An investment group invests $40,000
    in a certificate of deposit which pays
    12% annual interest, compounded
    quarterly. Find the value of this
    investment after 20 years.

3. _____

4. _____

5. To purchase additional park sites, a
    county treasurer invested $30,000 in
    an account which pays 8% annual
    interest, compounded quarterly. What
    is the value of the investment after
    5 years?

6. An employee invests $4000 in a
    corporate retirement account which
    pays 10% annual interest, compounded
    semi-annually. Find the value of this
    investment after 15 years.

5. _____

6. _____

7. An interior decorator deposited $4000
    in an account that pays 12% annual
    interest, compounded quarterly.
    a. What is the value of the investment
        in 15 years?
    b. How much interest was earned in
        the 15 years?

8. A business invests $80,000 in an
    account which pays 9% annual
    interest compounded quarterly.
    a. What is the value of the
        investment in five years?
    b. How much interest was earned
        in five years?

7. a. _____

   b. _____

8. a. _____

   b. _____

9. An investment of $6000 in an account
    which pays 12% annual interest
    compounded semi-annually, has a
    value of $34,460.90 after 15 years.
    a. What would have been the value
        if the 12% interest had been
        compounded daily over the
        15-year period?
    b. What is the difference in values of
        the investment after the 15 years?

10. A business has determined it will
    need $60,000 in five years for
    expansion. In an attempt to meet
    that goal, the business invests $40,000
    today in an account which pays 10%
    annual interest compounded quarterly.
    a. Find the value of the $40,000
        investment in five years.
    b. Will the business have enough
        money in the account for the
        planned expansion?

9. a. _____

   b. _____

10. a. _____

    b. _____

Name _____　　　　　　　　　　　Score _____

Solve.

1. A delicatessen is purchased for $260,000, and a down payment of $45,000 is made. Find the mortgage.

2. A beach house is purchased for $275,000, and a down payment of $95,000 is made. Find the mortgage.

1. _____

2. _____

3. A house is purchased for $72,300. The lender requires a down payment of 25%. Find the down payment.

4. A 2.5-acre parcel of land is purchased for $60,000. The lender requires a down payment of 20%. Find the down payment.

3. _____

4. _____

5. A marina is purchased for $175,000, and a down payment which is 18% of the purchase price is made. How much is the down payment?

6. An accountant makes a down payment of 20% of the $180,000 purchase price of an office building. How much is the down payment?

5. _____

6. _____

7. A credit union requires a borrower to pay $2\frac{1}{2}$ points for a loan. Find the loan origination fee for a loan of $80,000.

8. To purchase a small business, a person obtains a loan for $120,000. The loan origination fee is $4\frac{1}{2}$ points. Find the loan origination fee.

7. _____

8. _____

9. A farmer purchases some land for $150,000. The bank requires a down payment of 20%.
   a. Find the down payment.
   b. Find the mortgage.

10. A developer is selling a condominium for $88,000. A down payment of 10% is required.
   a. Find the down payment.
   b. Find the mortgage.

9. a. _____

b. _____

10. a. _____

b. _____

Name _____   Score _____

Solve. Use the Monthly Payment Table. Round to the nearest cent.

1. A self-storage business and a 20-year mortgage of $70,000 is obtained. The bank charges an annual interest rate of 16%. Find the monthly payment.

2. A group of investors obtained a loan of $200,000 to buy a small business. The monthly mortgage payment was based on 25 years at 17%. Find the monthly mortgage payment.

1. _____

2. _____

3. A company is considering purchasing a health club with a 25-year $350,000 mortgage at 18%. The treasurer has determined that the company can afford a monthly mortgage payment of $7000. can the company afford the monthly mortgage payment on the health club?

4. A couple interested in buying a home determines that they can afford a monthly mortgage payment of $685. Can they afford to buy a home with a 30-year $50,000 mortgage at 18% interest?

3. _____

4. _____

5. A county tax assessor has determined that the annual property tax on a $78,000 home is $765. Find the monthly property tax payment.

6. The annual property tax on a house is $680. Find the monthly property tax.

5. _____

6. _____

7. A home has a mortgage of $80,000 for 30 years at an annual interest rate of 17%.
   a. Find the monthly mortgage payment.
   b. During a month when $240.54 of the monthly mortgage payment is principal, how much of the payment is interest?

8. A factory which manufactures computer tables has a 20-year mortgage of $150,000 at an annual interest rate of 16%.
   a. Find the monthly mortgage payment.
   b. During a month when $268.88 of the monthly mortgage payment is principal, how much of the payment is interest?

7. a. _____

b. _____

8. a. _____

b. _____

9. A monthly mortgage on a home is $1320.40. The home owner must pay an annual property tax of $972. Find the total monthly payment for the mortgage and the property tax.

10. The monthly mortgage on a home is $1463.20. The owner must pay an annual property tax of $1171. Find the total monthly payment for the mortgage and the property tax.

9. _____

10. _____

Name _____   Score _____

Solve.

1. A car is purchased for $8500. A down payment of 12% is required. How much is the down payment?

2. A legal assistant has saved $970 to use as a down payment on a used car. The assistant's bank requires a down payment of 14% of the purchase price of a car. Does the assistant have enough saved to make a down payment on a car which costs $7850?

3. A carpenter purchases a used truck for $15,300 and must pay a sales tax of 4.5% of the purchase price. Find the sales tax.

4. A carpet salesperson buys a minivan to carry carpet samples. The purchase price of the minivan is $11,050 and a 4% sales tax is paid. How much is the sales tax?

5. A state charges a car license fee of 2% of the purchase price of a car. How much is the state car license fee for a car which costs $7595?

6. A license fee of 1.5% of the purchase price of a car is to be paid on a convertible costing $13,400. How much is the license fee for the car?

7. A pharmacist buys a car for $9550 with a down payment of $1750 and a sales tax of 3% of the purchase price.
   a. Find the sales tax.
   b. Find the total cost for the sales tax and the down payment.

8. An electrical contractor buys a $14,000 truck. A state license fee of $210 and a sales tax of 2.5% of the purchase price are required.
   a. Find the sales tax.
   b. Find the total cost for the sales tax and the license fee.

9. An airline employee buys a sports car for $24,000 and makes a down payment of 20% of the purchase price.
   a. Find the down payment.
   b. Find the amount financed.

10. A SUV is purchased for $10,500. A down payment of 15% is required. Find the amount financed.

1. _____

2. _____

3. _____

4. _____

5. _____

6. _____

7. a. _____

   b. _____

8. a. _____

   b. _____

9. a. _____

   b. _____

10. _____

Name _____   Score _____

Solve. Use the Monthly Payment Table. Round to the nearest cent.

1. A car loan of $5400 is financed
    through a credit union at an annual
    interest rate of 16% for 3 years. Find
    the monthly car payment.

2. A pickup truck is purchased by a
    furniture store owner and $9000 is
    financed through a bank at 15%
    interest for 48 months. Find the
    monthly payment.

1. _____

2. _____

3. It is estimated that when all costs of
    owning an economy car are considered,
    it costs $0.28 per mile to operate the
    car. Using this estimate, how much does
    it cost to operate a car during a year the
    car is driven 14,000 mi?

4. An estimate of the cost for care and
    maintenance of automobile tires is
    $0.016 per mile. Using this estimate,
    how much would it cost for care and
    maintenance during a year the car is
    driven 13,000 mi?

3. _____

4. _____

5. In a year when the total gasoline bill
    was $1680, the car was driven 12,000
    miles. What was the cost per miles
    for gasoline?

6. A car owner spent $1600 on gas, oil,
    and car insurance during a period
    when the car was driven 15,000 miles.
    Find the cost per mile for gas, oil, and
    car insurance.

5. _____

6. _____

7. During the year, $2100 was paid in
    monthly car payments, $1100 was spent
    on gasoline, and car insurance cost
    $330. Find the total cost for car payments,
    gasoline, and insurance for the year.

8. A car owner pays a monthly car
    payment of $154.60. During a month
    when $79.80 of the monthly payment
    is principal, how much of the payment
    is interest?

7. _____

8. _____

9. A used car is purchased for $6275, and
    a down payment of $1275 is made.
    The balance is financed for 3 years
    at an interest rate of 15%.
    a. Find the amount financed.
    b. Find the monthly car payment.

10. A used car is purchased for $12,000,
    and a down payment of $3000 is made.
    The balance is financed for 4 years
    at an annual interest rate of 16%.
    a. Find the amount financed.
    b. Find the monthly car payment.

9. a. _____

b. _____

10. a. _____

b. _____

11. A four-wheel drive truck is purchased
    for $9600, and a down payment of
    $2100 is made. The balance is financed
    for 3 years at an annual interest rate
    of 17%. Find the monthly truck payment.

12. A $8995 car is purchased with a down
    payment of $1945. The balance is
    financed for 4 years at an annual interest
    rate of 16%. Find the monthly car
    payment.

11. _____

12. _____

Name _____   Score _____

Solve. Round to the nearest cent.

1. A part time sales clerk earns an hourly wage of $9.85. How much does the sales clerk earn during a 24-hour work week?

2. A checker in a food store earns $7.20 per hour. How much does the checker earn in a 40-hour work week?

1. _____

2. _____

3. A junior executive for a marketing research firm receives an annual salary of $43,800. How much does the executive receive per month?

4. A legal assistant receives $25,500 annually. How much does the assistant earn each month?

3. _____

4. _____

5. A brick layer's hourly wage is $24.25. For working overtime, the brick layer earns double time. What is the brick layer's hourly wage for working overtime?

6. A golf pro receives a commission of 20% for selling a set of golf clubs. Find the commission earned by the golf pro for selling a set of golf clubs which cost $390.

5. _____

6. _____

7. A sales representative for a computer store receives a commission of 11% on the weekly sales. Find the commission earned during a week when sales were $4100.

8. An agent for a leasing company receives a commission of 2.5% for leasing office space. Find the commission received by the agent for leasing an office space for $72,000.

7. _____

8. _____

9. A roofer receives $2.50 per square yard to install roofing. How much does the roofer receive for installing 180 square yards of roofing?

10. An acoustic consultant received a contract for $3600. The consultant spent 45 hours working on the project. Find the consultant's hourly wage.

9. _____

10. _____

11. A video technician's hourly wage is $14.60. For working overtime, the technician receives double time.
    a. What is the technician's hourly wage for working overtime?
    b. How much does the technician earn for working 12 hours of overtime?

12. A company which sells medical equipment pays its sales executives a commission of 12% of all sales over $120,000. During one year, a sales executive sold $440,000 worth of medical equipment.
    a. Find the amount of sales over $120,000.
    b. Find the commission earned by the sales executive.

11. a. _____

   b. _____

12. a. _____

   b. _____

Name _____ Score _____

Solve.

1. A nurse had a checking account balance of $504.37 before writing a check for $59.42. What is the current account balance?

2. A hotel manager had a checking account balance of $433.62 before making a deposit of $134.74. What is the current checking account balance?

   1. _____

   2. _____

3. The business checking account for a grocery store showed a balance of $2625.36. What is the balance in the account after making a deposit of $528.06?

4. An automobile rental firm had a balance of $3542.87 in its checking account. What is the balance in the account after writing a check for $1198.17?

   3. _____

   4. _____

5. A food broker had a checking account balance of $435.86 before writing a check for $38.44 and making a deposit of $170. Find the current checkbook balance.

6. A warranty clerk had a checking account balance of $279.54 before writing one check for $28.36 and another check for $19.15. Find the current checkbook balance.

   5. _____

   6. _____

7. An assistant manager had a checkbook balance of $218.74 before making a deposit of $145 and writing a check for $336.47. Is there enough money in the account for the bank to pay the check?

8. A receptionist had a checkbook balance of $135.87 before making a deposit of $260 and writing a check for $415. Is there enough money in the account for the bank to pay the check?

   7. _____

   8. _____

9. An inventory clerk's checkbook balance is $834.51. The clerk wants to purchase a TV for $495 and a used sofa for $275. Is there enough money in the account to make the two purchases?

10. A medical assistant has a current checkbook balance of $909.70. The assistant wants to purchase an organ for $725 and a stereo amplifier for $215.60. Is there enough money in the account to make the purchases?

   9. _____

   10. _____

Name _____　　Score

Solve.

1.　Your checkbook shows a balance of $417.25. The bank statement does not show a deposit of $172.54, and checks for $45.82 and $204.53 have not been cashed. What balance does the bank statement show?

2.　Your checkbook shows a balance of $115.28. The bank statement does not show deposits of $96.82 and $112.58, and checks for $12.39 and $79.65 have not been cashed. What balance does the bank statement show?

1. _____

2. _____

3.　Your checkbook shows a balance of $202.53. The bank statement does not show a deposit of $116.16, and checks for $49.85 and $189.12 have not been cashed. What balance does the bank statement show?

4.　Your checkbook shows a balance of $523.69. The bank statement does not show a deposit of $117.13, and checks for $59.16 and $325 have not been cashed. What balance does the bank statement show?

3. _____

4. _____

5.　Your checkbook shows a balance of $810.63. The bank statement does not show a deposit of $210.15, and checks for $112.95 and $315.42 have not been cashed. What balance does the bank statement show?

6.　Your checkbook shows a balance of $608.07. The bank statement does not show a deposit of $98.58, and checks for $69.54 and $142.69 have not been cashed. What balance does the bank statement show?

5. _____

6. _____

7.　Your checkbook shows a balance of $1025.67. The bank statement does not show a deposit of $405.14, and checks for $129.35 and $375 have not been cashed. What balance does the bank statement show?

8.　Your checkbook shows a balance of $790.39. The bank statement does not show a deposit of $516.80, and checks for $217.56, $28.95 and $187.60 have not been cashed. What balance does the bank statement show?

7. _____

8. _____

9.　Your checkbook shows a balance of $1468.72. The bank statement does not show a deposit of $851, and checks for $110.81, $350 and $94.26 have not been cashed. What balance does the bank statement show?

10.　Your checkbook shows a balance of $1620.87. The bank statement does not show a deposit of $920.76, and checks for $268.71, $127.42 and $67.50 have not been cashed. What balance does the bank statement show?

9. _____

10. _____

Name   Score

The pictograph shows the number of iPods purchased in a metropolitan area during a 4-month period.

September   ▸▸ ▸▸ ▸▸ ▸▸ ▸
October   ▸▸ ▸▸ ▸
November   ▸▸ ▸▸ ▸▸
December   ▸▸ ▸▸ ▸▸ ▸▸ ▸▸ ▸▸ ▸▸ ▸▸
             ▸▸ = 100 iPods

1. Find the total number of iPods purchased during the 4-month period.

2. How many more iPods were purchased in December than in October?

    1. _____

    2. _____

3. The number of iPods purchased in September represents what percent of the total number of iPods purchased during the 4-month period?

4. Find the ratio of the number of iPods purchased in November to the number of iPods purchased in September.

    3. _____

    4. _____

The pictograph in the figure below is based on a survey of 500 college students who were asked for their favorite pizza location.

Corner Pizza Shop   ●●●●
Major Chain (eat in)   ●
Major Chain (delivery) ●●◖
Grocery store (frozen) ●◖
                        ● = 10%

5. Find the number of students who preferred the Corner Pizza Shop.

6. Find the number of students who preferred Major Chain – delivery.

    5. _____

    6. _____

7. What is the difference between the Major Chain–eat in, and the Major Chain – delivery?

8. Find the ratio of the number who preferred Major Chain – delivery to the Grocery Store – frozen.

    7. _____

    8. _____

Name _____   Score _____

The circle graph below shows the distribution of an employee's gross monthly income of $4000.

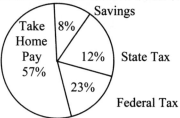

1.   Find the employee's take-home pay.   2.   Find the amount placed into savings.   1. _____

2. _____

3.   Find the amount taken out for state and federal taxes.   4.   What is the ratio of state tax to federal tax?   3. _____

4. _____

The circle graph below shows the distribution of sales at a fast food restaurant. Sales total $1,600,000.

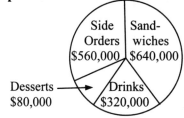

5.   What is the ratio of the sale of sandwiches to the total sales?   6.   What is the ratio of the sale of drinks to the total sales?   5. _____

6. _____

7.   What is the ratio of the sale of side orders to the total sales?   8.   What is the ratio of the sale of drinks and desserts to the sale of sandwiches and side orders?   7. _____

8. _____

Name   Score

The bar graph below shows the annual salaries of the managers of a chain of electronics stores in five states.

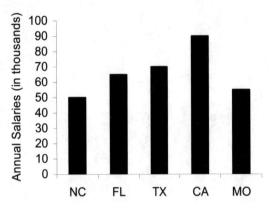

1. How much does the Texas manager earn?

2. How much does the Missouri manager earn?

1. _____

2. _____

3. How much does the Florida manager earn?

4. What is the difference between the salaries of the managers from California and North Carolina?

3. _____

4. _____

The double-bar graph below shows the number of flat screen TVs sold by a chain of electronics stores for the last 5 months of 2003 and 2004.

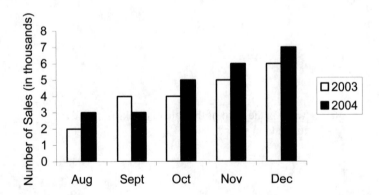

5. Find the number of TVs sold in September, 2004.

6. In 2003, during which month were sales lowest?

5. _____

6. _____

7. What is the difference between the December sales for 2003 and 2004?

8. What is the total August sales for 2003 and 2004?

7. _____

8. _____

Name   Score

The broken-line graph below shows the monthly sales for a clothing store for each of the last six months of a year.

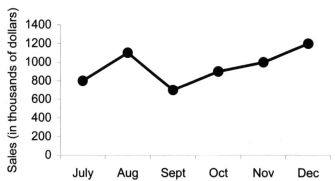

1.   What were the sales for October?   2.   What were the sales for December?   1.   _____

                                                                                                2.   _____

3.   During what month were the sales   4.   During what month were the sales the   3.   _____
       the lowest?   highest?

                                                                                                4.   _____

The broken-line graph below shows the quarterly automobile sales for 2003 and 2004.

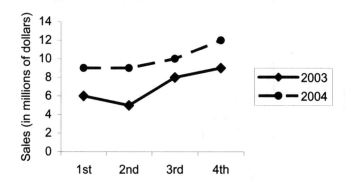

5.   Find the sales for the fourth quarter   6.   Find the sales for the second quarter of   5.   _____
       of 2004.   2003.

                                                                                                6.   _____

7.   Find the difference between the   8.   Find the combined sales for the   7.   _____
       first-quarter sales for 2003 and 2004.   third and fourth quarters of 2004.

                                                                                                8.   _____

Name   Score

The fuel usage of 100 cars was measured by a research group. The results are recorded in the histogram below.

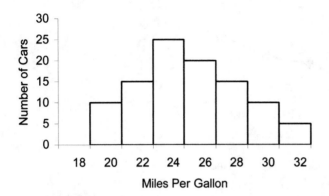

1. Find the number of cars which get between 24 and 26 miles per gallon.

2. Find the ratio of the number of cars which get between 30 and 32 miles per gallon to the total number of cars.

3. Find the number of cars which get 24 or more miles per gallon.

4. Find the ratio of the number of cars which get between 18 and 22 miles per gallon to the number that get between 26 and 30 miles per gallon.

1. _____

2. _____

3. _____

4. _____

The hourly wages of the 100 employees of a company are recorded in the histogram below.

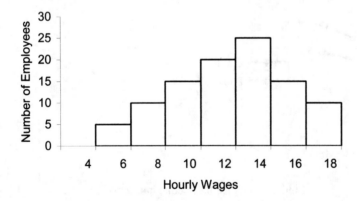

5. Find the number of employees whose hourly wage is between $6 and $10.

6. Find the ratio of the number of employees whose hourly wage is between $12 and $14 to the total number of employees.

7. Find the number of employees whose hourly wages is between $8 and $14.

8. How many employees earn $12 or more per hour?

5. _____

6. _____

7. _____

8. _____

Name _____   Score _____

A radio rating service surveyed 105 families to find the number of hours they listened to the radio. The results are recorded in the figure below.

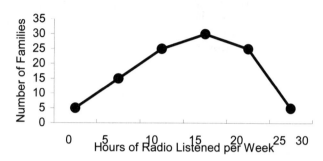

1. How many families listened between 10 and 15 hours a week?

2. What is the ratio of the number of families who listened between 20 and 25 hours a week to the total number in the survey?

1. _____

2. _____

3. How many families listened between 20 and 30 hours a week?

4. What is the ratio of the number of families who listened 15 or more hours a week to the total number in the survey?

3. _____

4. _____

A real estate company sold 100 homes during the last three months. The selling prices are recorded in the figure below.

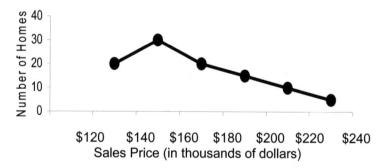

5. How many homes sold for between $140,000 and $160,000?

6. Find the ratio of the number of homes which sold for between $120,000 and $140,000 to the total number of homes sold during the three months.

5. _____

6. _____

7. How many homes sold for between $160,000 and $240,000?

8. How many homes sold for between $120,000 and $180,000?

7. _____

8. _____

Name _____ Score _____

Solve.

1. The prices of a scientific calculator at five stores were $16.25, $15.75, $16.15, $16.50, and $16.95. Find the mean price of the calculator.

2. A student received grades of 83, 89, 85, 91, and 92 on five mathematics exams. Find the mean grade of the student's mathematics exams.

1. _____

2. _____

3. The six sales representatives for an advertising agency received weekly bonuses of $345, $275, $190, $221, $335, and $260. Find the mean bonus.

4. A number of pizzas sold in five different stores over a three-day period was 212, 246, 205, 252, and 245. Find the mean number of pizzas sold per store during this period of time.

3. _____

4. _____

5. The prices of identical CD clock radios at each of five stores were $33.25, $39.00, $36.75, $36.00, and $37.50. Find the median price of the CD clock radio.

6. The number of miles driven during each of five days of a business trip was 107, 96, 151, 103, and 99. Find the median number of miles driven.

5. _____

6. _____

7. The hourly wages for seven job classifications at a company are $7.63, $10.43, $10.09, $7.59, $8.45, $7.47, and $8.38. Find the median hourly wage.

8. The ages of the seven most recently hired employees at a fast food store are 22, 41, 19, 21, 20, 26, and 29. Find the median age.

7. _____

8. _____

9. The number of responses to a discount coupon for a carpet cleaner during a six-day period was 35, 29, 33, 37, 28 and 26. What is the mode of the data?

10. The scores on eight math exams at a job placement service were 79, 93, 95, 69, 93, 96, 88, and 75. What is the mode of the data?

9. _____

10. _____

Name   Score

The ages of the 300 accountants who passed the certified public accountant (CPA) exam at one test center were recorded. The box-and-whiskers plot below shows the distribution of their scores.

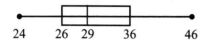

24   26 29   36   46

1.   What is the youngest age?   2.   What is the greatest oldest age?   1. _____

                                                                                          2. _____

3.   What is the first quartile?   4.   What is the third quartile?   3. _____

                                                                                          4. _____

5.   What is the median?   6.   What is the range?   5. _____

                                                                                          6. _____

7.   What is the interquartile range?   8.   How many of the accountants were   7. _____
                                              older than 36?

                                                                                          8. _____

9.   How many of the accountants were   10.   How many accountants are represented   9. _____
      younger than 29?   in each quartile?

                                                                                          10. _____

11.   What percent of the accountants were 12.   What percent of the accountants were   11. _____
      younger than 36?   older than 46?

                                                                                          12. _____

Name   Score

Solve.

1. Two dice are rolled. What is the probability that the sum of the dots on the upwards faces is 4?

2. Two dice are rolled. What is the probability that the sum of the dots on the upwards faces is 9?

1. _____

2. _____

3. Two dice are rolled. What is the probability that the sum of the dots on the upwards faces is greater than 1?

4. A coin is tossed 3 times. What is the probability that the outcomes of the tosses consist of two tails and one head?

3. _____

4. _____

5. Each of the letters of the word *MISSISSIPPI* is written on a card, and the cards are placed in a hat. One card is drawn at random from the hat. What is the probability that the card has the letter *S* on it?

6. Each of the letters of the word *MISSISSIPPI* is written on a card, and the cards are placed in a hat. One card is drawn at random from the hat. What is the probability that the card has the letter *P* on it?

5. _____

6. _____

7. Which has a greater probability, drawing a 5, 6, or 10 from a deck of cards or drawing a diamond?

8. In a psychology class, a set of exams earned the following grades: 6 A's, 9 B's, 16 C's, 5 D's, and 3 F's. If a single student's exam is chosen from this class, what is the probability that it received an A?

7. _____

8. _____

9. Six purple marbles, four orange marbles, and eight blue marbles are placed in a bag. One marble is chosen at random. What is the probability that the marble chosen is purple?

10. Seven purple marbles, five orange marbles, and three blue marbles are placed in a bag. One marble is chosen at random. What is the probability that the marble chosen is orange?

9. _____

10. _____

Name _____ Score _____

Convert.

1.   5 ft = _____ in.

2. $8\frac{1}{2}$ ft = _____ in.

3. $9\frac{1}{3}$ ft. = _____ in.

4. $12\frac{2}{3}$ ft = _____ in.

5.   60 in. = _____ ft

6.   54 in. = _____ ft

7.   72 in. = _____ ft

8.   70 in. = _____ ft

9. $3\frac{1}{3}$ yd = _____ ft

10. $4\frac{2}{3}$ yd = _____ ft

11.   30 ft = _____ yd

12.   18 ft = _____ yd

13.   15 ft = _____ yd

14. $5\frac{1}{2}$ yd = _____ in.

15.   72 in. = _____ yd

16.   120 in. = _____ yd

17.   96 in. = _____ yd

18.   3 mi = _____ ft

19. $4\frac{1}{2}$ mi = _____ ft

20.   5 mi = _____ ft

21. $2\frac{1}{3}$ mi = _____ ft

22.   140 in. = _____ ft

23. $7\frac{1}{2}$ ft = _____ in.

24. $2\frac{1}{4}$ yd = _____ in.

25. $5\frac{1}{2}$ ft = _____ in.

26.   10,560 ft = _____ mi

27.   7290 ft = _____ mi

1. _____

2. _____

3. _____

4. _____

5. _____

6. _____

7. _____

8. _____

9. _____

10. _____

11. _____

12. _____

13. _____

14. _____

15. _____

16. _____

17. _____

18. _____

19. _____

20. _____

21. _____

22. _____

23. _____

24. _____

25. _____

26. _____

27. _____

Name   Score

Perform the arithmetic operation.

1.   3200 ft = _____ yd _____ ft   2.   7000 ft = _____ mi _____ ft   1.   _____

                                                                                      2.   _____

3.   160 in. = _____ ft _____ in.   4.   8000 ft = _____ mi _____ ft   3.   _____

                                                                                      4.   _____

5.   2000 ft = _____ yd _____ ft   6.   8 ft 13 in.   5.   _____
                                                + 2 ft 7 in.
                                                                                      6.   _____

7.   11 ft 15 in.   8.   10 ft 3 in.   7.   _____
     + 7 ft 8 in.   − 6 ft 8 in.
                                                                                      8.   _____

9.   5 ft 10 in.   10. $5\frac{1}{3}$ ft ×6   9.   _____
        ×   6
                                                                                      10. _____

11. $4\frac{2}{3}$ ft ×9   12. $8\frac{1}{3}$ ft ×12   11. _____

                                                                                      12. _____

13. $6\overline{)9\text{ ft 6 in.}}$ 14. $5\frac{1}{4}$ ft $+ 3\frac{1}{2}$ ft 13. _____

                                                                                      14. _____

15. $6\frac{1}{3}$ ft $+ 9\frac{3}{4}$ ft   16. $7\frac{5}{6}$ ft $+ 11\frac{1}{2}$ ft   15. _____

                                                                                      16. _____

17. 10 ft $- 8\frac{1}{2}$ ft   18. $24\frac{1}{2}$ ft $- 19\frac{1}{4}$ ft 17. _____

                                                                                      18. _____

19. $12\frac{3}{4}$ yd $- 4\frac{5}{8}$ yd   20.   2 mi 2100 ft   19. _____
                                                   + 3 mi 3900 ft
                                                                                      20. _____

Name _____ Score _____

Solve.

1. Four pieces of steel, each $1\frac{3}{8}$ in. thick are stacked together. Find the resulting thickness of the four pieces of steel.

2. A piece of plastic pipe $4\frac{1}{2}$ feet long is cut into four equal pieces. How long is each piece?

1. _____

2. _____

3. Find the length of the shaft.

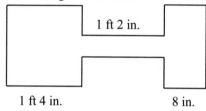

1 ft 2 in.

1 ft 4 in.   8 in.

4. Find the missing dimension.

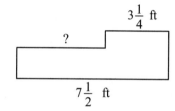

$3\frac{1}{4}$ ft

?

$7\frac{1}{2}$ ft

3. _____

4. _____

5. Forty-two yards of crepe paper were used for decorating. How many feet of crepe paper were used?

6. You purchased 28 feet of window stripping to winterize your house. How many inches of window stripping did you buy?

5. _____

6. _____

7. A picture is 2 ft 8 in. wide and 1 ft 9 in. high. Find the length of the framing needed to put around the picture.

8. Thirty concrete block each 9 in. long, are laid end to end to make the foundation for a wall. Find the length of the wall in feet.

7. _____

8. _____

9. You use 46 ft of a roll of copper tubing containing 40 yd of tubing. How many feet of tubing are left on the roll?

10. Your back yard is being fenced. The dimensions are $11\frac{1}{2}$ ft, $8\frac{2}{3}$ yd, $12\frac{1}{3}$ yd, and $9\frac{1}{2}$ yd. The fencing costs $7 per yard. Find the cost to fence in the back yard.

9. _____

10. _____

Name _____ Score _____

Convert.

1. 3 lb = _____ oz

2. 32 oz = _____ lb

3. 5 tons = _____ lb

4. $4\frac{1}{4}$ tons = _____ lb

5. 8000 lb = _____ tons

6. 9200 lb = _____ tons

7. $\frac{3}{5}$ tons = _____ lb

8. $\frac{5}{8}$ tons = _____ lb

9. $6\frac{1}{5}$ tons = _____ lb

10. 14 lb = _____ oz

11. 6400 lb = _____ tons

12. 3600 lb = _____ tons

13. 100 oz = _____ lb

14. 90 oz = _____ lb

15. 300 oz = _____ lb

16. $3\frac{1}{10}$ tons = _____ lb

17. $5\frac{2}{5}$ tons = _____ lb

18. 4500 lb = _____ tons

19. $2\frac{3}{5}$ tons = _____ lb

20. 192 oz = _____ lb

21. $9\frac{3}{4}$ lb = _____ oz

22. 168 oz = _____ lb

23. 62 oz = _____ lb

24. 80 oz = _____ lb

25. $7\frac{3}{4}$ lb = _____ oz

26. $4\frac{3}{8}$ lb = _____ oz

27. $\frac{2}{5}$ tons = _____ lb

1. _____
2. _____
3. _____
4. _____
5. _____
6. _____
7. _____
8. _____
9. _____
10. _____
11. _____
12. _____
13. _____
14. _____
15. _____
16. _____
17. _____
18. _____
19. _____
20. _____
21. _____
22. _____
23. _____
24. _____
25. _____
26. _____
27. _____

Name　　　　　　　　　　　　　　　　　　　　　　　　　　　　　　Score

Perform the arithmetic operation.

1.　7000 lb = _____ tons _____ lb

2.　76 oz = _____ lb _____ oz

3.　90 oz = _____ lb _____ oz

4.　100 oz = _____ lb _____ oz

5.　140 oz = _____ lb _____ oz

6.　　8 lb 6 oz
　　+ 7 lb 9 oz

7.　　11 lb 12 oz
　　+ 6 lb 6 oz

8.　　2 tons 900 lb
　　+ 4 tons 1200 lb

9.　　5 tons 600 lb
　　+ 9 tons 800 lb

10.　10 tons 1600 lb
　　+ 5 tons 500 lb

11.　　5 tons 1600 lb
　　− 2 tons 1800 lb

12.　　9 tons 1000 lb
　　− 3 tons 1500 lb

13.　$6\frac{1}{2}$ oz $\times 8$

14.　$5\frac{3}{8}$ lb $\times 4$

15.　　$5\frac{1}{4}$ oz
　　+ $3\frac{3}{4}$ oz

16.　　$9\frac{5}{8}$ oz
　　+ $3\frac{1}{4}$ oz

17.　$3\overline{)2\text{ lb 7 oz}}$

18.　$5\overline{)2\text{ tons 100 lb}}$

1. _____

2. _____

3. _____

4. _____

5. _____

6. _____

7. _____

8. _____

9. _____

10. _____

11. _____

12. _____

13. _____

14. _____

15. _____

16. _____

17. _____

18. _____

105

Name　　　　　　　　　　　　　　　　　　　　　　　　　　　　Score

Solve.

1.　A brick weighs $2\frac{1}{2}$ lb. Find the weight of a load of 300 bricks.

2.　A case of tomatoes contains 24 cases of $10\frac{1}{2}$-ounce cans. Find the weight of the case of tomatoes.

3.　A box of one brand of detergent weighs 40 oz. Find the weight of a 12-package case of detergent.

4.　A box of one brand of powdered milk weighs $4\frac{3}{8}$ lb and another box $2\frac{9}{16}$ lb. Find the difference in the weight of the two boxes of detergent.

5.　A 9-by-9-inch tile weighs 8 oz. Find the weight in pounds of a package of 96 tiles.

6.　Find the weight in pounds of 48 bars of soap. Each bar weighs 9 ounces.

7.　Hamburger meat weighing 20 lb is equally divided and placed into 8 containers. How much hamburger is in each container?

8.　Find the cost of a package of chicken breast weighing 3 lb 4 oz if the price is $2.20 per pound.

9.　Two books were mailed at the rate of $0.15 per ounce. The books weighed 1 lb 2 oz and 1 lb 15 oz. Find the total cost of mailing the books.

10.　A gourmet food store buys 18 lb of cheese for $27.36. The cheese is cut and packaged and sold in 12-ounce packages for $2.40 each. Find the mark-up on the 18 lb of cheese.

1. _____

2. _____

3. _____

4. _____

5. _____

6. _____

7. _____

8. _____

9. _____

10. _____

Name   Score

Convert.

1. 24 fl oz = _____ c

2. 2 c = _____ fl oz

3. 12 c = _____ pt

4. 7 c = _____ pt

5. $2\frac{1}{2}$ pt = _____ c

6. 10 pt = _____ qt

7. 20 qt = _____ gal

8. 12 qt = _____ gal

9. 6 gal = _____ qt

10. 9 pt = _____ qt

11. $6\frac{1}{2}$ qt = _____ pt

12. 5 gal = _____ qt

13. 4 qt = _____ c

14. 7 qt = _____ c

15. 120 fl oz = _____ c

16. 9 c = _____ fl oz

17. 20 c = _____ pt

18. $6\frac{1}{2}$ pt = _____ c

19. 24 pt = _____ qt

20. $1\frac{1}{4}$ gal = _____ qt

21. 40 fl oz = _____ pt

22. 10 gal = _____ qt

23. 9 gal = _____ pt

24. 6 c = _____ fl oz

25. 48 fl oz = _____ pt

26. 32 qt = _____ gal

27. $5\frac{1}{2}$ pt = _____ qt

1. _____
2. _____
3. _____
4. _____
5. _____
6. _____
7. _____
8. _____
9. _____
10. _____
11. _____
12. _____
13. _____
14. _____
15. _____
16. _____
17. _____
18. _____
19. _____
20. _____
21. _____
22. _____
23. _____
24. _____
25. _____
26. _____
27. _____

Name _____   Score _____

Perform the arithmetic operation.

1.   7 pt = _____ qt _____ pt

2.   11 pt = _____ qt _____ pt

1. _____

2. _____

3.   3 qt 1 pt
    + 1 qt 1 pt

4. $2\frac{1}{2}$ pt ×6

3. _____

4. _____

5. $4\frac{1}{2}$ gal ×3

6.   2 gal 1 qt
    + 3 gal 2 qt

5. _____

6. _____

7.   4 gal 1 qt
    − 1 gal 3 qt

8.   6 c 2 fl oz
    − 2 c 5 fl oz

7. _____

8. _____

9.   5 gal 3 qt
    − 2 gal 3 qt

10.   3 c 2 fl oz
    + 2 c 7 fl oz

9. _____

10. _____

11.   5 gal
    − 3 gal 1 qt

12.   4 gal 2 qt
    − 1 gal 3 qt

11. _____

12. _____

13. $3\frac{1}{2}$ qt ×4

14. $3\frac{1}{4}$ gal ×8

13. _____

14. _____

15.   4 qt
    − 1 qt 1 pt

16.   5 c
    − 2 c 5 fl oz

15. _____

16. _____

17.   4 c 6 fl oz
    + 3 c 4 fl oz

18.   3 gal 2 qt
    + 1 gal 3 qt

17. _____

18. _____

Name _____　　　　Score _____

Solve.

1. If a serving contains 1 cup, how many servings can be made from 11 gallons of punch?

2. A breakfast bar sold 88 cartons of orange juice in one day. Each carton contained 1 cup of juice. How many quarts of orange juice were sold that day?

1. _____

2. _____

3. One hundred twelve people attended the opening of the art exhibit. Assume that each person drank a cup of punch. How many gallons of punch were served?

4. A recipe calls for 10 ounces of tomato sauce. How many cups of tomato sauce will be needed if the recipe is tripled?

3. _____

4. _____

5. Forty-eight people are going ice skating. Assume that each person will drink 2 c of hot chocolate. How many gallons of hot chocolate should be prepared?

6. A college student changed the oil in a compact car 6 times during the year. Each oil change required $3\frac{1}{2}$ qt of oil. How many gallons of oil did the student use in the six oil changes?

5. _____

6. _____

7. A can of pineapple juice contains 28 oz. Find the number of pints of pineapple juice in a case of 12 cans.

8. A cross-country skier is carrying 6 quarts of water. Water weighs $8\frac{1}{3}$ lb per gallon. Find the weight of water that is carried by the skier.

7. _____

8. _____

9. Brand A cranberry juice costs $1.35 for 1 qt. Brand B costs $1.12 for 24 oz of cranberry juice. Find the more economical brand.

10. A drugstore bought 6 qt of shampoo and repackaged it in 6 fluid ounce bottles. The shampoo cost $35.50 and each 6 fluid ounce bottle was sold for $2.25. How much profit was made on the shampoo?

9. _____

10. _____

Name   Score

Convert.

1. 91 days = _____ weeks

2. $6\frac{1}{4}$ h = _____ min

3. 3600 min = _____ days

4. 15,300 s = _____ h

5. 2220 s = _____ min

6. 6 days = _____ h

7. 1176 h = _____ weeks

8. 45 weeks = _____ days

9. 1020 min = _____ h

10. 18 h = _____ s

11. 90 h = _____ days

12. $5\frac{1}{2}$ days = _____ min

13. 4 weeks = _____ h

14. 16 min = _____ s

1. _____

2. _____

3. _____

4. _____

5. _____

6. _____

7. _____

8. _____

9. _____

10. _____

11. _____

12. _____

13. _____

14. _____

Name _____   Score _____

Solve.

1. Convert 45 BTU to foot-pounds.

2. Convert 3000 BTU to foot-pounds.

3. Convert 550 BTU to foot-pounds

4. Convert 30,000 BTU to foot-pounds

5. Find the energy required to lift 2500-pound car a distance of 8 ft.

6. Six tons are lifted 5 ft. Find the energy required in foot-pounds.

7. Four tons are lifted 6 ft. Find the energy required in foot-pounds.

8. Eight tons are lifted 12 ft. Find the energy required in foot-pounds.

9. Find the energy required for a 150-lb person to climb a 4000 ft high mountain.

10. Find the energy required for a motor to lift 700 lb through a distance of 12 ft.

11. A furnace is rated at 40,000 BTU per hour. How many foot-pounds of energy are released by the furnace in one hour?

12. A furnace is rated at 75,000 BTU per hour. How many foot-pounds of energy are released by the furnace in one hour?

13. Find the amount of energy in foot-pounds given off when 1 lb of fuel oil is burned. One pound of fuel oil gives off 15,000 BTU of energy when burned.

14. A plumber carries 8-pound sections of pipe up a 10-foot flight of stairs. How many foot-pounds of energy are required to carry 12 sections of pipe up the stairs?

1. _____

2. _____

3. _____

4. _____

5. _____

6. _____

7. _____

8. _____

9. _____

10. _____

11. _____

12. _____

13. _____

14. _____

Name _____   Score _____

Solve.

1. Convert 6600 $\frac{\text{ft-lb}}{\text{s}}$ to horsepower.

2. Convert 4950 $\frac{\text{ft-lb}}{\text{s}}$ to horsepower.

    1. _____

    2. _____

3. Convert 10 hp to foot-pounds per second.

4. Convert 15 hp to foot-pounds per second.

    3. _____

    4. _____

5. Find the power in foot-pounds per second needed to raise 1800 lb a distance of 20 ft in 15 s.

6. Find the power in foot-pounds per second needed to raise 2000 lb a distance of 18 ft in 20 s.

    5. _____

    6. _____

7. Find the power in foot-pounds per second needed to raise 16,000 lb a distance of 30 ft in 40 s.

8. Find the power in foot-pounds per second needed to raise 4500 lb to a height of 20 ft in 45 s.

    7. _____

    8. _____

9. Find the power in foot-pounds per second needed to raise 1800 lb to a height of 24 ft in 36 s.

10. A motor has a power of 13,200 $\frac{\text{ft-lb}}{\text{s}}$. Find the horsepower of the motor.

    9. _____

    10. _____

11. A motor has a power of 5500 $\frac{\text{ft-lb}}{\text{s}}$. Find the horsepower of the motor.

12. A motor has a power of 13,750 $\frac{\text{ft-lb}}{\text{s}}$. Find the horsepower of the motor.

    11. _____

    12. _____

13. A motor has a power of 17,600 $\frac{\text{ft-lb}}{\text{s}}$. Find the horsepower of the motor.

14. A motor has a power of 8800 $\frac{\text{ft-lb}}{\text{s}}$. Find the horsepower of the motor.

    13. _____

    14. _____

Name _____   Score _____

Convert.

1. 84 mm = _____ cm   2. 57.3 mm = _____ cm   3. 84.2 km = _____ m   1. _____

                                                                                            2. _____

                                                                                            3. _____

4. 196 cm = _____ m   5. 72.8 cm = _____ m   6. 6.42 m = _____ cm   4. _____

                                                                                            5. _____

                                                                                            6. _____

7. 83 cm = _____ mm   8. 97 mm = _____ cm   9. 5716 m = _____ km   7. _____

                                                                                            8. _____

                                                                                            9. _____

10. 23.128 km = _____ m   11. 10.8 km = _____ m   12. 82.5 cm = _____ m   10. _____

                                                                                            11. _____

                                                                                            12. _____

13. 9.63 m = _____ cm   14. 126 cm = _____ mm   15. 243 mm = _____ cm   13. _____

                                                                                            14. _____

                                                                                            15. _____

16. 176.6 mm = _____ cm   17. 5713 m = _____ km   18. 4.218 km = _____ m   16. _____

                                                                                            17. _____

                                                                                            18. _____

19. 9.63 m = _____ cm   20. 46.9 mm = _____ cm   21. 196 cm = _____ mm   19. _____

                                                                                            20. _____

                                                                                            21. _____

22. 7539 m = _____ km   23. 4.218 km = _____ m   24. 9 m 35 cm = _____ cm   22. _____

                                                                                            23. _____

                                                                                            24. _____

25. 84 cm 4 mm = _____ mm 26. 97 km 51 m = _____ m 27. 17 cm 9 mm = _____ mm 25. _____

                                                                                            26. _____

                                                                                            27. _____

Name   Score

Solve. Round to the nearest hundredth.

1. Find the amount of wood needed to build a form around the patio.

2. Find the missing dimension in centimeters.

3. An aluminum frame 7 m 56 cm long is cut into four equal pieces. Find the length of each piece.

4. Three pieces of weather stripping are cut from a 20-meter roll. The three pieces measure 2 m 20 cm, 3 m 60 cm, and 4 m 80 cm. How much of the weather stripping is left after the three cuts are made?

5. A letter carrier walked 2 km 300 m in the morning and 3 km 250 m in the afternoon. This is 1 km 150 m less than a second carrier walked. How far did the second letter carrier walk?

6. Four pieces of coaxial cable are cut from a 100-meter roll. The four pieces are 9 m 50 cm, 6 m 80 cm, 12 m 70 cm, and 21 m 60 cm. How much of the cable is left after the four cuts are made?

7. A living room is 5 m 40 cm wide and 6 m 70 cm long. Find the length of molding needed to put around the top edge of the four walls.

8. Underground telephone lines are being places from the main line to three houses. The three pieces measure 8 m 50 cm, 16 m 70 cm, and 12 m 90 cm. Find the average length of the three lines.

9. A stereo cabinet 2 m 75 cm long has three shelves. Find the cost of the shelves when the price of lumber is $10.60 per meter.

10. During the week you swam 2 km 500 m, 3 km, 3 km 400 m, and 4 km 100 m. Find the average distance swum each of the four days.

1. _____

2. _____

3. _____

4. _____

5. _____

6. _____

7. _____

8. _____

9. _____

10. _____

Name   Score

Convert.

1. 6309 g = _____ kg   2. 254 mg = _____ g   3. 58 mg = _____ g   1. _____

                                                                                                2. _____

                                                                                                3. _____

4. 0.154 kg = _____ g   5. 0.56 g = _____ mg   6. 2754 g = _____ kg   4. _____

                                                                                                5. _____

                                                                                                6. _____

7. 3248 mg = _____ g   8. 0.345 g = _____ mg   9. 3.91 kg = _____ g   7. _____

                                                                                                8. _____

                                                                                                9. _____

10. 1639 mg = _____ g   11. 0.0228 g = _____ mg   12. 0.98 g = _____ mg   10. _____

                                                                                                11. _____

                                                                                                12. _____

13. 975 g = _____ mg   14. 86 mg = _____ g   15. 5.4 kg = _____ g   13. _____

                                                                                                14. _____

                                                                                                15. _____

16. 0.72 kg = _____ g   17. 854 g = _____ kg   18. 634 g = _____ kg   16. _____

                                                                                                17. _____

                                                                                                18. _____

19. 38 mg = _____ g   20. 171 mg = _____ g   21. 7.9 kg = _____ g   19. _____

                                                                                                20. _____

                                                                                                21. _____

22. 0.123 kg = _____ g   23. 0.15 g = _____ mg   24. 1347 g = _____ mg   22. _____

                                                                                                23. _____

                                                                                                24. _____

25. 1.856 kg = _____ g   26. 11 g 780 mg = _____ mg   27. 317 g 84 mg = _____ mg   25. _____

                                                                                                26. _____

                                                                                                27. _____

Name   Score

Solve.

1.   A student weighs 64 kg 280 g. How much does the student weigh in kilograms after gaining 2 kg 120 g?

2.   A 9-by-9 inch tile weighs 350 g. Find the weight in kilograms of a box containing 72 tiles.

1.   _____

2.   _____

3.   A shopper bought cheese weighing 650 g, 720 g, 870 g, and 500 g. Find the total weight in kilograms of the cheese.

4.   A brick weighs 450 g. Find the weight in kilograms of a load of 600 bricks.

3.   _____

4.   _____

5.   How many VCRs weighing 12 kg each can be placed on a shelf with a maximum load limit of 100 kg?

6.   Find the cost of a ham weighing 4 kg 225 g if the price per kilogram is $2.98. Round to the nearest cent.

5.   _____

6.   _____

7.   Five hundred grams of fertilizer are used for each of the 600 trees in an apple orchard. At $1.50 per kilogram of fertilizer, how much does it cost to fertilize the apple orchard.

8.   A store buys 20 kg of coffee for $80. The store packages the coffee in 250-gram bags and sells them for $3.00 per bag. Find the profit on the 20 kg of coffee.

7.   _____

8.   _____

9.   It is recommended that 1 kg of fertilizer be used for every 15 trees in an orange grove. Find the amount of fertilizer required for 1800 trees.

10.   An airline charges $2.50 for each kilogram or part of a kilogram over 40 kg of luggage weight. How much extra must be paid for three pieces of luggage weighing 24 kg 400 g, 17 kg 500 g, and 15 kg?

9.   _____

10.   _____

Name _____ Score _____

Add.

1. 5.8 ml = _____ L

2. 0.16 ml = _____ cm^3

3. 0.065 cm^3 = _____ ml

4. 67 cm^3 = _____ L

5. 1038 cm^3 = _____ L

6. 0.536 L = _____ cm^3

7. 1.65 L = _____ cm^3

8. 2 L 138 ml = _____ cm^3

9. 3 L 325 ml = _____ cm^3

10. 4 L 50 ml = _____ cm^3

11. 5 L 738 ml = _____ cm^3

12. 9 L 269 ml = _____ cm^3

13. 11 L 28 ml = _____ cm^3

14. 3.31 kl = _____ L

15. 0.075 kl = _____ L

16. 2347 L = _____ kl

17. 2700 ml = _____ L

18. 3.2 ml = _____ L

19. 6.84 L = _____ kl

20. 2076 cm^3 = _____ L

21. 0.083 L = _____ cm^3

22. 937 ml = _____ cm^3

23. 2 L 679 ml = _____ cm^3

24. 4 L 38 ml = _____ cm^3

25. 71 cm^3 = _____ L

26. 1 L 36 ml = _____ L

27. 5 L 254 ml = _____ L

1. _____
2. _____
3. _____
4. _____
5. _____
6. _____
7. _____
8. _____
9. _____
10. _____
11. _____
12. _____
13. _____
14. _____
15. _____
16. _____
17. _____
18. _____
19. _____
20. _____
21. _____
22. _____
23. _____
24. _____
25. _____
26. _____
27. _____

Name   Score

Solve.

1. A concession stand at the fair sold 1038 medium soft drinks. Each medium soft drink cup contains 540 ml. How many liters of soft drink were sold?

2. A motorist bought 40 liters of gasoline. The cost of the gasoline was $15.40. Find the cost of one liter of gasoline.

1. _____

2. _____

3. There are 48 bottles in a case of shampoo. Each bottle contains 450 ml of shampoo. How many liters of shampoo are in one case?

4. A bottle of steak sauce contains 50 ml of tomato sauce. How many liters of tomato sauce are used when preparing 240 bottles of steak sauce?

3. _____

4. _____

5. A food processor used 125 ml of vinegar in each jar of pickles. How many liters of vinegar are used when 600 jars of pickles are prepared?

6. A health clinic buys 6 L of flu vaccine. How many people can be immunized if each person receives 4 cm^3 of vaccine?

5. _____

6. _____

7. Sixty-two percent of a cologne is distilled water. Find the amount of water in 15 L of cologne.

8. One hundred twenty people are going to attend a piano recital. Assuming that each person drinks 250 ml of punch, how many liters of punch should be prepared?

7. _____

8. _____

9. Thirty-four liters of ketchup are bought and then repackaged in 680 milliliter containers. Thirty-four containers of ketchup are sold. How many 680-ml containers are still in stock?

10. Eight liters of hair conditioner are bought for $60. The hair conditioner is repackaged in 125-milliliter bottles and sold for $2.85 per bottle. Find the profit on the 8 L of hair conditioner.

9. _____

10. _____

Name   Score

Solve.

1. How many Calories can be omitted from your diet in four weeks by omitting 350 Calories per day?

2. You omit one pat of butter at lunch and dinner for 28 days. If a pat of butter contains 50 Calories, how many Calories will you omit from your diet?

1. _____

2. _____

3. You consumed 420 Calories for breakfast, 930 Calories for lunch, and 1380 Calories for dinner. How many Calories did you consume during the day?

4. You are on a diet limiting your Calorie intake to 2000 Calories per day. You consume 445 Calories for breakfast. How many more Calories can you consume during the remainder of the day?

3. _____

4. _____

5. Find the cost of 720 kilowatt hours of electricity at $0.105 per kilowatt hour.

6. A portable TV is rated at 90 watts. The TV is used for 31 h one week. How many kilowatts of energy are used?

5. _____

6. _____

7. A microwave oven uses 500 watts of energy. How many watt-hours of energy are used to cook a 6-kilogram turkey for 2 h?

8. A 1300-watt dishwasher is used an average of 3.5 h per week. How many kilowatt-hours of energy are used each week?

7. _____

8. _____

9. An electric clothes dryer uses 4800 watts of energy. The dryer is used for 24 h one month. At a cost of 9.8¢ per kilowatt-hour, how much does it cost to use the dryer for that month?

10. A house is insulated to save energy. The house used 310 kW h of electrical energy per month before insulation and saved 62 kW h of energy per month after insulation. What percent decrease does this represent?

9. _____

10. _____

Name   Score

Convert. Round to the nearest hundredth.

1. Convert a 200-yard race to meters.

2. Find the weight in kilograms of a 187-pound person.

1. _____

2. _____

3. Find the number of liters in 6 gal of coffee.

4. Find the number of liters in 15.6 gal of gasoline.

3. _____

4. _____

5. Find the number of milliliters in 3 cups of milk.

6. The winning pole vault at a track meet was 18 ft 4 in. Convert this height to meters.

5. _____

6. _____

7. Express 60 mi/h in kilometers per hour.

8. Express 59 mi/h in kilometers per hour.

7. _____

8. _____

9. Canadian bacon costs $2.90 per pound. Find the cost per kilogram.

10. Grapes cost $1.49 per pound. Find the cost per kilogram.

9. _____

10. _____

11. The cost of oil for an outboard motor is $4.80 per gallon. Find the cost per liter.

12. Redwood stain costs $12.00 per gallon. Find the cost per liter.

11. _____

12. _____

13. Riding a bicycle requires 265 Calories per hour. How many pounds could be lost by biking 2 h each days for 8 days if no extra Calories were consumed? (3500 Calories is equivalent to 1 lb.)

14. The price of low-fat milk is $2.05 per gallon. Find the cost per liter to the nearest cent.

13. _____

14. _____

15. The distance from Los Angeles to Atlanta is 2200 mi. Convert this distance to kilometers.

16. The distance from San Francisco to Miami is 3075 mi. Convert this distance to kilometers.

15. _____

16. _____

120

Name _____ Score _____

Convert. Round to the nearest hundredth.

1.   Convert a 300-meter race to feet.

2.   Find the weight in pounds of a 76-kilogram person.

   1. _____

   2. _____

3.   Find the number of gallons in 8 L of antifreeze.

4.   Your height is 1.72 m. Find your height in inches.

   3. _____

   4. _____

5.   Find the distance of a 2500-meter race in feet.

6.   Find the weight in ounces of 500 g of cereal.

   5. _____

   6. _____

7.   How many gallons does a 64-liter tank hold?

8.   Find the width of a 40 mm piece of tape in inches.

   7. _____

   8. _____

9.   A bottle of ketchup contains 906 ml. Find the number of pints in 906 ml.

10.   Express 76 km/h in miles per hour.

   9. _____

   10. _____

11.   Diesel fuel costs 32.5¢ per liter. Find the cost per gallon.

12.   A ham costs $4.30 per kilogram. Find the cost per pound.

   11. _____

   12. _____

13.   Jet fuel costs 40.5¢ per liter. Find the cost per gallon.

14.   The cost of ice cream is $1.60 per liter. Find the cost per gallon to the nearest cent.

   13. _____

   14. _____

15.   Swimming uses approximately 480 Calories per hour. How many hours of swimming is necessary to lose 1 lb? (3500 Calories is equivalent to 1 lb.)

16.   An egg contains approximately 75 Calories. How many pounds can be lost in 39 days by omitting one egg from a daily diet? (3500 Calories is equivalent to 1 lb.)

   15. _____

   16. _____

Name
Score

Represent the quantity by a signed number.

1. A gain of $265

2. A temperature that is 5° below zero

3. Stock down $5\frac{3}{4}$ points

4. A cliff 5480 ft above sea level

1. _____

2. _____

3. _____

4. _____

Graph the number on the number line.

5. 4, –4

6. 0, 1

7. –2, 1

8. –3, –4

5. __(see graph)__

6. __(see graph)__

7. __(see graph)__

8. __(see graph)__

Place the correct symbol, < or >, between the two numbers.

9. –7   0

10. –4   –3

11. 5   –6

12. –14   –24

13. $4\frac{1}{9}$ $-5\frac{2}{3}$

14. $-10\frac{1}{3}$ $-10\frac{1}{7}$

9. _____

10. _____

11. _____

12. _____

13. _____

14. _____

Write the given numbers from smallest to largest.

15. 6, –15, –8, 2

16. 9, –5, 0, 7

17. 3, 0, –9, 12

15. _____

16. _____

17. _____

Name _____ Score _____

Find the opposite number.

1. 9

2. 3

3. -15

1. _____

2. _____

3. _____

Evaluate.

4. $-\left|65\right|$

5. $\left|-10\right|$

6. $-\left|-3\right|$

4. _____

5. _____

6. _____

7. $\left|-0.6\right|$

8. $\left|2\frac{6}{7}\right|$

9. $-\left|-19\right|$

7. _____

8. _____

9. _____

10. $\left|-28.1\right|$

11. $-\left|-\frac{5}{8}\right|$

12. $-\left|9.7\right|$

10. _____

11. _____

12. _____

Place the correct symbol <, =, or > between the two numbers.

13. $\left|-14\right|$ $\left|17\right|$

14. $-\left|4.03\right|$ $\left|-5\right|$

15. $\left|35.4\right|$ $-\left|36\right|$

13. _____

14. _____

15. _____

16. $-\left|1.5\right|$ $\left|-1.5\right|$

17. $\left|-4\right|$ $\left|4\right|$

18. $-\left|-9\right|$ $-\left|-15\right|$

16. _____

17. _____

18. _____

Write the given numbers in order from smallest to largest.

19. $-\left|-1\right|,\ -3,\ \left|-4\right|,\ \left|6\right|$ **20.** $\left|-10\right|,\ 7,\ \left|-3\right|,\ -\left|9\right|$ **21.** $\left|2\right|,\ \left|-5\right|,\ -6,\ -\left|10\right|$

19. _____

20. _____

21. _____

Name

Score

Add.

1. 6 + 2

2. −5 + 3

3. −13 + 7

4. 44 + (−71)

5. −25 + (−16)

6. 186 + (−98)

7. 4 + 9 + (−10)

8. −14 + (−3) + 8

9. 13 + (−28) + 7

10. −30 + (−22)

11. −42 + 28 + 14

12. 29 + (−11) + (−4)

13. −5 + 9 + (−18)

14. −7 + (−12) + 8

15. 10 + (−4) + (−19)

16. 186 + (−17)

17. −292 + 351

18. −421 + (−109)

19. −12 + 37 + (−15)

20. 41 + (−8) + (−16)

21. 32 + (−23) + 11

22. −6 + (−15) + (−9) + 18

23. 4 + (−13) + 7 + (−17)

24. −21 + 30 + (−7) + (−12)

1. _____

2. _____

3. _____

4. _____

5. _____

6. _____

7. _____

8. _____

9. _____

10. _____

11. _____

12. _____

13. _____

14. _____

15. _____

16. _____

17. _____

18. _____

19. _____

20. _____

21. _____

22. _____

23. _____

24. _____

Name   Score

Subtract.

1. $12 - 8$	**2.** $4 - 15$	**3.** $-5 - 16$	**1.** _____
			2. _____
			3. _____
4. $42 - (-37)$	**5.** $-53 - (-37)$	**6.** $-108 - 95$	**4.** _____
			5. _____
			6. _____
7. $-6 - 17 - (-11)$	**8.** $-16 - (-18) - (-13)$	**9.** $25 - 13 - (-7)$	**7.** _____
			8. _____
			9. _____
10. $-42 - 23 - 9$	**11.** $79 - 12 - 53$	**12.** $-15 - (-33) - (-27)$	**10.** _____
			11. _____
			12. _____
13. $-3 - 4 - (-9)$	**14.** $-12 - (-15) - 2$	**15.** $18 - (-7) - (-3)$	**13.** _____
			14. _____
			15. _____
16. $-8 - (-42)$	**17.** $-29 - 24$	**18.** $10 - 29$	**16.** _____
			17. _____
			18. _____
19. $-7 - (-15) - 13$	**20.** $8 - 23 - (-11)$	**21.** $-14 - (-3) - 9$	**19.** _____
			20. _____
			21. _____
22. $-4 - 15 - (-28) - 5$	**23.** $23 - (-19) - 12 - 6$	**24.** $-5 - (-14) - (-9) - (-1)$	**22.** _____
			23. _____
			24. _____

Name _____   Score _____

Solve.

1. Find the temperature after a rise of 9°C from –9°C.

2. Find the temperature after a rise of 4°C from –15°C.

1. _____

2. _____

3. During a game of Scrabble, Dan had a score of 70 points before his opponent used all the tiles, subtracting a score of 11 from Dan's total. What was Dan's score after his opponent ended the game?

4. During a game of Scrabble, Jean had a score of 115 points before she used all her tiles, entitling her to add 16 points to her score. What was Jean's score after she ended the game?

3. _____

4. _____

5. Find the temperature after a decrease of 10°F from 3°F.

6. Find the temperature after a decrease of 24°F from 52°F.

5. _____

6. _____

7. In a Minnesota city, the average nighttime temperature in January was –28°F and the average daytime temperature can reach 14°F. Find the difference between these average temperatures.

8. In a California city, the average nighttime temperature in July was –78°F and the average daytime temperature can reach 105°F. Find the difference between these average temperatures.

7. _____

8. _____

9. The elevation for Mt. Everest is 8850 meters and the elevation for the Dead Sea is –411 meters. What is the difference in elevation between Mt. Everest and the Dead Sea?

10. The elevation for Mt. McKinley is 5642 meters and the elevation for Death Valley is –28 meters. What is the difference in elevation between Mt. McKinley and Death Valley?

9. _____

10. _____

Name   Score

Multiply.

1. $-4(8)$ **2.** $8(-7)$ **3.** $-4(-9)$ **1.** _____

                                                                                             2. _____

                                                                                             3. _____

4. $-9\times(-11)$ **5.** $0\times(-13)$ **6.** $-17(-29)$ **4.** _____

                                                                                             5. _____

                                                                                             6. _____

7. $3\times8\times(-7)$ **8.** $-9\times(-7)\times8$ **9.** $18\times(-3)\times6$ **7.** _____

                                                                                             8. _____

                                                                                             9. _____

10. $-8\times(-12)\times(-4)$ **11.** $-16\times4\times10$ **12.** $30\times(-5)\times0$ **10.** _____

                                                                                             11. _____

                                                                                             12. _____

13. $6\cdot(-13)$ **14.** $-13(-4)$ **15.** $-8(-15)$ **13.** _____

                                                                                             14. _____

                                                                                             15. _____

16. $23(-5)$ **17.** -6×12 **18.** $9(-14)$ **16.** _____

                                                                                             17. _____

                                                                                             18. _____

19. $-2\times(-8)\times4$ **20.** $3\times(-10)\times(-3)$ **21.** $-4\times(-2)\times(-10)$ **19.** _____

                                                                                             20. _____

                                                                                             21. _____

Name   Score

Divide. Round to the nearest hundredth.

1. $18 \div (-6)$	**2.** $-54 \div 6$	**3.** $-35 \div (-5)$	**1.** _____
			2. _____
			3. _____
4. $-37 \div 8$	**5.** $35 \div (-7)$	**6.** $-40 \div 4$	**4.** _____
			5. _____
			6. _____
7. $-96 \div (-8)$	**8.** $-54 \div 0$	**9.** $-85 \div (-16)$	**7.** _____
			8. _____
			9. _____
10. $217 \div (-30)$	**11.** $-642 \div (-25)$	**12.** $-963 \div 54$	**10.** _____
			11. _____
			12. _____
13. $141 \div (-3)$	**14.** $0 \div (-30)$	**15.** $-174 \div (-6)$	**13.** _____
			14. _____
			15. _____
16. $84 \div (-7)$	**17.** $-924 \div 11$	**18.** $-280 \div (-4)$	**16.** _____
			17. _____
			18. _____
19. $-56 \div 4$	**20.** $-32 \div (-8)$	**21.** $910 \div (-13)$	**19.** _____
			20. _____
			21. _____

Name

Score

Solve.

1. The combined scores of the top eight golfers in a tournament equaled –24 (24 under par). What was the average score of the eight golfers?

2. The daily high temperatures during one week were recorded as follows: –10°C, –4°C, 1°C, –11°C, –16°C, –7°C, and –2°C. Find the average daily high temperature for the week.

1. _____

2. _____

3. The daily low temperatures during one week were recorded as follows: –20°C, –7°C, –18°C, –15°C, –23°C, –13°C, and –2°C. Find the average daily low temperature for the week.

4. The combined scores of the top six golfers in a tournament equaled –42 (42 under par). What was the average score of the top six golfers?

3. _____

4. _____

5. To discourage guessing on a multiple-choice exam, an instructor graded the test by giving 6 points for a correct answer, –2 point for an answer left blank, and -4 points for an incorrect answer. How many points did a student score who answered 21 questions correctly, answered 6 questions incorrectly, and left 4 questions blank?

6. The value of a stock can increase and decrease every day. The daily increase or decrease for a stock during one week was recorded as follows: –1.05, –2.50, 0.74, –0.38, 0.49. Find the average increase or decrease for the stock for the week.

5. _____

6. _____

7. The value of a stock can increase and decrease every day. The daily increase or decrease for a stock during one week was recorded as follows: –6.27, 0.99, 0.75, –0.10, 0.53. Find the average increase or decrease for the stock for the week.

8. To discourage guessing on a multiple-choice exam, an instructor graded the test by giving 7 points for a correct answer, –3 point for an answer left blank, and -7 points for an incorrect answer. How many points did a student score who answered 21 questions correctly, answered 6 questions incorrectly, and left 3 questions blank?

7. _____

8. _____

Name _____   Score _____

Add.

1. $-\dfrac{1}{4}+\left(-\dfrac{5}{6}\right)$

2. $\dfrac{7}{9}+\left(-\dfrac{1}{3}\right)$

3. $-\dfrac{4}{5}+1\dfrac{3}{7}$

4. $\dfrac{1}{6}+\left(-\dfrac{8}{9}\right)+\left(-\dfrac{1}{4}\right)$

5. $-\dfrac{5}{8}+\left(-\dfrac{7}{12}\right)+\left(-\dfrac{1}{2}\right)$

6. $-2\dfrac{1}{8}+\dfrac{2}{3}+\left(-4\dfrac{4}{9}\right)$

7. $7.4+(-3.8)$

8. $-6.52+(-10.8)$

9. $-16.013+4.215$

10. $-12.1+(-5.8)+2.31$

11. $6.05+(-0.17)$

12. $6.214-(-4.61)$

Subtract.

13. $-2\dfrac{1}{3}-\left(-\dfrac{7}{8}\right)$

14. $\dfrac{3}{4}-\dfrac{5}{12}-\left(-\dfrac{1}{5}\right)$

15. $-\dfrac{7}{22}-\left(-\dfrac{2}{11}\right)-\left(-\dfrac{1}{4}\right)$

16. $4\dfrac{1}{5}-\dfrac{4}{15}-\left(-3\dfrac{2}{3}\right)$

17. $-12.45-17.82$

18. $-23.061-(-14.005)$

19. $8.3-(-10.64)$

20. $-3.272-4.1$

21. $17.5-8.36-(0.19)$

1. _____

2. _____

3. _____

4. _____

5. _____

6. _____

7. _____

8. _____

9. _____

10. _____

11. _____

12. _____

13. _____

14. _____

15. _____

16. _____

17. _____

18. _____

19. _____

20. _____

21. _____

Name _____ Score _____

Multiply.

1. $-\dfrac{5}{6}\times\dfrac{3}{10}$

2. $-\dfrac{7}{12}\times\left(-\dfrac{4}{9}\right)$

3. $\dfrac{3}{8}\times\left(-\dfrac{5}{8}\right)$

4. $-2\dfrac{3}{5}\times\left(-\dfrac{10}{13}\right)$

5. $3\dfrac{3}{4}\times\left(-3\dfrac{1}{5}\right)$

6. $-1\dfrac{7}{9}\times2\dfrac{1}{2}$

7. $-5.4(-3.1)$

8. $-8.2(11.7)$

9. $8.5\times(-15.6)$

1. _____

2. _____

3. _____

4. _____

5. _____

6. _____

7. _____

8. _____

9. _____

Divide.

10. $\dfrac{1}{9}\div\left(-\dfrac{1}{8}\right)$

11. $-\dfrac{5}{7}\div\dfrac{4}{7}$

12. $-\dfrac{3}{5}\div\left(-\dfrac{9}{10}\right)$

13. $-\dfrac{3}{4}\div1\dfrac{7}{8}$

14. $-3\dfrac{2}{3}\div\left(-6\dfrac{3}{5}\right)$

15. $8\dfrac{1}{6}\div\left(-4\dfrac{2}{3}\right)$

16. $-28.53\div(-9)$

17. $-9.41\div8$

18. $0\div(-7.35)$

10. _____

11. _____

12. _____

13. _____

14. _____

15. _____

16. _____

17. _____

18. _____

131

Name   Score

Solve.

1. On February 6, the temperature in
    Bradford, PA was 7.32°F. On February 7,
    the temperature in Bradford, PA was
    −32.67°F. Find the difference between
    the temperatures on these two days.

2. On January 19, the temperature in
    Buffalo, NY was 5.69°F. On January 20,
    the temperature was −16.54°F. Find the
    difference in temperature.

1. _____

2. _____

3. The lowest temperature on a south-
    Western desert was −29.8°F. The
    highest temperature was 131.6°F.
    Find the difference between these
    two extremes.

4. On Friday, the closing price of a
    share of a tech stock was $8.07. The
    change in the closing price from the
    previous day was −$0.11. Find the
    closing price on Thursday.

3. _____

4. _____

5. On Tuesday, the closing price of a
    share of a pharmaceutical stock was
    $157.63. The change in the closing
    price from the previous day was −$0.48.
    Find the closing price on Monday.

6. At noon the temperature was 15.27°F
    and at midnight it fell to −10.85°F.
    How many degrees did the temperature
    fall?

5. _____

6. _____

7. On Thursday, the closing price of a
    share of oil stock was $52.76. The
    change in the closing price from the
    previous day was −$0.81. Find the
    closing price on Wednesday.

8. On Wednesday, the closing price of
    a share of a utility stock was $76.58.
    The change in the closing price from
    the previous day was −$0.74. Find the
    closing price on Tuesday.

7. _____

8. _____

Name _____   Score _____

Write the number in scientific notation.

1. 420,000

2. 0.0000079

3. 3,620,000,000

4. 82,000,000,000

5. 0.000000081

6. 0.000000154

7. 0.0000000066

8. 738,500,000

1. _____

2. _____

3. _____

4. _____

5. _____

6. _____

7. _____

8. _____

Write the number in decimal notation.

9. 4.63×10^{-5}

10. 6.95×10^{7}

11. 2.576×10^{10}

12. 1.29×10^{-8}

13. 9.11×10^{6}

14. 5.73×10^{8}

15. 3.78×10^{-4}

16. 7.14×10^{-7}

9. _____

10. _____

11. _____

12. _____

13. _____

14. _____

15. _____

16. _____

Name   Score

Simplify.

1. $9 \div 3 + 7$

2. $2 - 15 \div 5$

3. $7 - (3^2) \times 5$

4. $(-4)^2 - (8)^2 - (-9)$

5. $14 \div 7 - 6 \div 2$

6. $(-5)^2 \times 2 \div (9 + 1)$

7. $9 \times 2 - 4 \times 5 + 6 \times 3 + 7 - 3$

8. $-5 \times (-3)^2 \times 2 \div 3 - (-10)$

9. $2^2 \times (3 - 4) \div 2 + 5 - 8 \times 2$

10. $(-6)^2 \times (6 - 4)^2 - (-12) \div 4$

11. $(3.4)^2 - 7.2 \times 0.8$

12. $6.4 \times 8 \div (-3.2)$

13. $2.9 \times (-4.7) - 5$

14. $(7.5 - 3.4) \times (-4.6)$

15. $(-0.8)^2 \times 1.5 - 3.9$

16. $\left(-\dfrac{3}{4}\right)^2 \div \dfrac{3}{8}$

1. _____

2. _____

3. _____

4. _____

5. _____

6. _____

7. _____

8. _____

9. _____

10. _____

11. _____

12. _____

13. _____

14. _____

15. _____

16. _____

Name _____   Score _____

Evaluate the variable expression when $a = 2$, $b = 3$, and $c = 4$.

1. $ab + c$

2. $2a + b$

3. $a + 3c$

4. $3a + 4c$

5. $ac - b$

6. $b^2 + a$

7. $c - ab^2$

8. $b^2 - a$

9. $a^2 - b$

10. $abc - c^2$

11. $-b^2$

12. $(-a)^2$

13. $(-c)^2$

14. $c^2 + 2b$

15. $c - (a - b)$

16. $b - ab$

17. $3ab - c^2$

18. $3a^2 - c$

19. $ab^2 - c^2$

20. $a(b^2 - c^2)$

21. $bc \div (ac)$

22. $c^2 - a^2 + b^2$

23. $c^2 - (a^2 + b)$

24. $2a - 3b - c^2$

25. $a^2 + b^2 + c^2$

26. $a^2 - b^2 + c^2$

27. $a^2 - ab + c^2$

1. _____

2. _____

3. _____

4. _____

5. _____

6. _____

7. _____

8. _____

9. _____

10. _____

11. _____

12. _____

13. _____

14. _____

15. _____

16. _____

17. _____

18. _____

19. _____

20. _____

21. _____

22. _____

23. _____

24. _____

25. _____

26. _____

27. _____

Name   Score

Simplify.

1. $6a + 8a$

2. $7x + 4x$

3. $6y - 14y$

4. $-15mn + 8mn$

5. $6x^2 + 7x^2$

6. $6x - 3 + 4x$

7. $t + 9t - 6t$

8. $-6y + 8y - y$

9. $7uv - 13uv + uv$

10. $2y^2 - xy + 4y^2$

11. $8x^2 - 3 - 2x^2$

12. $5w - 6u + 7w$

13. $-ab - 5ab - 8ab$

14. $6x^2 - x^2 - 5y^2$

15. $-7xy - 6y + 5xy$

16. $-9ab - 4a + 3ab$

17. $6x^2 - 8y - x^2 + 7y$

18. $7y - 3z - y + 3z$

19. $11y^2 - 3y + 4y^2 - 4y$

20. $4x - y - 8x + 6y$

21. $6w - v - 10w + 6v$

22. $6m + 10n - 3m + 4n$

23. $2z - 10y - 5z + 6y$

24. $-7ab + 5ac + ab - ac$

25. $-3x^2 - 2x - 8x^2 - 11x^2$

26. $4a^2 - 7ab - a^2 - ab$

27. $-x^2 - 4x - 10x^2 + 11x$

1. _____

2. _____

3. _____

4. _____

5. _____

6. _____

7. _____

8. _____

9. _____

10. _____

11. _____

12. _____

13. _____

14. _____

15. _____

16. _____

17. _____

18. _____

19. _____

20. _____

21. _____

22. _____

23. _____

24. _____

25. _____

26. _____

27. _____

Name _____   Score _____

Simplify.

1. $3(x+2)$

2. $5(m+4)$

3. $(y-2)7$

4. $-3(a+3)$

5. $-4(a+5)$

6. $9(x-y)$

7. $-2(x-1)$

8. $5(3x-1)$

9. $4(3x+8)$

10. $3(2m-5)$

11. $-2(w-5)$

12. $-4(v-9)$

13. $4(a-b)$

14. $8(m-3)$

15. $7(2a-1)$

16. $3x+2(x-6)$

17. $6x-2(x-4)$

18. $8x-3(x-7)$

19. $-2m+2(m+3)$

20. $6m+3(m+5)$

21. $-6x+5(x+7)$

22. $7y-2(y-3)+7$

23. $4-3(a+3)+4a$

24. $6x+3(x+1)+7x$

25. $9x+2(x-2)+5x$

26. $-6y+2(y-3)-y$

27. $x-3(2-x)-3x$

1. _____
2. _____
3. _____
4. _____
5. _____
6. _____
7. _____
8. _____
9. _____
10. _____
11. _____
12. _____
13. _____
14. _____
15. _____
16. _____
17. _____
18. _____
19. _____
20. _____
21. _____
22. _____
23. _____
24. _____
25. _____
26. _____
27. _____

Name _____   Score _____

Solve.

1. Is 3 a solution of $4x = 12$?

2. Is 5 a solution of $3x = 18$?

3. Is 4 a solution of $2x + 3 = 11$?

4. Is 3 a solution of $2 - 3x = 7$?

5. Is -3 a solution of $5x + 9 = 2x$?

6. Is 4 a solution of $16 - x = 3x$?

7. Is -1 a solution of $3x - 1 = x - 3$?

8. Is 6 a solution of $3x - 7 = 5 + x$?

9. Is 5 a solution of $3 + x = 13 - x$?

10. Is -4 a solution of $4x + 7 = 13 - x$?

11. Is 2 a solution of $5 - 2x = 7 - x$?

12. Is -1 a solution of $x^2 - 3x - 4 = 0$?

13. Is 2 a solution of $x^2 - 2x + 1 = (x-1)^2$?

14. Is 4 a solution of $x^2 + 3x + 2 = 6$?

15. Is -2 a solution of $x^2 - 5x - 1 = 9 - 2x$?

16. Is -5 a solution of $x(x-3) = x^2 + 15$?

17. Is 3 a solution of $x(x-1) = x^2 + 3$?

18. Is -5 a solution of $x^2 - 2x - 1 = 9 - 5x$?

19. Is -7 a solution of $x^2 + 7x = 9 - 5x$?

20. Is $-\dfrac{1}{3}$ a solution of $5x - 1 = 1 - x$?

1. _____

2. _____

3. _____

4. _____

5. _____

6. _____

7. _____

8. _____

9. _____

10. _____

11. _____

12. _____

13. _____

14. _____

15. _____

16. _____

17. _____

18. _____

19. _____

20. _____

Name _____

Score _____

Solve.

1. $x + 5 = 11$

2. $5 + n = 8$

3. $x + 5 = 1$

4. $w + 10 = 3$

5. $x - 2 = -6$

6. $x + 7 = 7$

7. $t - 5 = -3$

8. $v - 6 = -2$

9. $x - 4 = -1$

10. $1 - x = 0$

11. $5 + y = 0$

12. $x - 11 = 6$

13. $y - 3 = 7$

14. $x + 3 = -8$

15. $t - 4 = -9$

16. $x + 2 = -7$

17. $t - 1 = -8$

18. $w + 8 = -3$

19. $z - 1 = 1$

20. $x + 6 = -5$

21. $x + \dfrac{3}{4} = \dfrac{1}{4}$

22. $x - \dfrac{3}{7} = -\dfrac{1}{7}$

23. $y + \dfrac{4}{9} = -\dfrac{2}{9}$

24. $\dfrac{5}{8} + y = -\dfrac{1}{8}$

25. $x - 3.2 = 7.8$

26. $x + 1.6 = 8$

27. $x - 2.9 = -9.9$

1. _____
2. _____
3. _____
4. _____
5. _____
6. _____
7. _____
8. _____
9. _____
10. _____
11. _____
12. _____
13. _____
14. _____
15. _____
16. _____
17. _____
18. _____
19. _____
20. _____
21. _____
22. _____
23. _____
24. _____
25. _____
26. _____
27. _____

Name   Score

Solve.

1. $2x = 8$

2. $5x = 25$

3. $-6x = 12$

1. _____

2. _____

3. _____

4. $-5t = 40$

5. $54 = 9y$

6. $63 = -9y$

4. _____

5. _____

6. _____

7. $-20 = -5y$

8. $-35 = 5y$

9. $\dfrac{x}{5} = 4$

7. _____

8. _____

9. _____

10. $\dfrac{x}{3} = 9$

11. $\dfrac{n}{3} = -6$

12. $\dfrac{x}{6} = -5$

10. _____

11. _____

12. _____

13. $-\dfrac{x}{5} = 2$

14. $-\dfrac{m}{8} = 3$

15. $-\dfrac{1}{4}x = -3$

13. _____

14. _____

15. _____

16. $-\dfrac{1}{3}y = -2$

17. $\dfrac{4}{7}x = 8$

18. $\dfrac{2}{3}v = -4$

16. _____

17. _____

18. _____

19. $\dfrac{2}{5}x = -8$

20. $-\dfrac{3}{10}w = 15$

21. $-8 = -\dfrac{2}{3}z$

19. _____

20. _____

21. _____

22. $\dfrac{5}{6}x = 20$

23. $\dfrac{3}{8}x = -24$

24. $-30 = -\dfrac{5}{6}y$

22. _____

23. _____

24. _____

25. $-12 = \dfrac{3}{4}t$

26. $\dfrac{3}{7}x = -18$

27. $\dfrac{5}{8}a - \dfrac{3}{8}a = 7$

25. _____

26. _____

27. _____

Name   Score

Solve.

Use the formula $P = R - C$, where P is the profit, R is the revenue, and C is the amount spent for one week.

1.   The profit for the week was $17,000.   2.   The revenue for the week was $16,000.   1. _____
     The amount spent was $14,250. Find   The amount spent was $11,200. Find
     the revenue for the week.   the profit for the week.

                                                                                                  2. _____

Use the formula $S = R - D \cdot R$, where S is the sale price, R is the regular price, and D is the discount rate.

3.   During a clearance sale, all items are   4.   The discount rate is 25%. The regular   3. _____
     discounted 30%. Find the regular price   price of a sweater is $60. Find the
     of a suit on sale for $126.   sale price.

                                                                                                  4. _____

Use the formula $A = P + I \cdot P$, where A is the value of the investment in one year, P is the original investment, and I is the interest rate for the investment.

5.   Find the interest rate for an original   6.   An investor purchased $10,000 worth   5. _____
     investment of $6000 which had a value   of gold bullion. One year later the
     of $7500 after one year.   gold was worth $12,000. Find the
                                                        interest rate for the investment.

                                                                                                  6. _____

Use the formula $S = CY + B$, where S is the total salary, C is the commission rate, Y is the value of the sales completed, and B is the base salary.

7.   Find the total salary of a real estate   8.   Find the base salary of a sales   7. _____
     agent whose base salary is $1000,   representative whose total salary
     commission rate is 2%, and who sold   was $4000, commission rate was 4%,
     property valued at $250,000.   and who had sold merchandise valued
                                                        at $80,000.
                                                                                                  8. _____

Name _____ Score _____

Solve.

1. $3x - 1 = 8$ 2. $5x - 8 = 27$ 3. $7x + 9 = -5$

4. $3x + 4 = 22$ 5. $5x + 9 = -6$ 6. $7 + 2x = 9$

7. $15 + 7x = 36$ 8. $6 - x = -1$ 9. $5 - 4x = -3$

10. $3 - 2x = 15$ 11. $7 - 4x = -21$ 12. $4 - 6x = 10$

13. $2x + 10 = 0$ 14. $3x - 21 = 0$ 15. $9 - 5x = 14$

16. $-3x - 22 = -1$ 17. $10x - 14 = 16$ 18. $7x + 9 = 2$

19. $4x + 7 = -5$ 20. $6x - 110 = 10$ 21. $-2x + 9 = -5$

22. $-3x + 13 = -2$ 23. $9 - 2x = 5$ 24. $11x - 7 = 26$

25. $5x + 9 = 4$ 26. $-6x + 17 = -1$ 27. $6 - 3x = 12$

1. _____

2. _____

3. _____

4. _____

5. _____

6. _____

7. _____

8. _____

9. _____

10. _____

11. _____

12. _____

13. _____

14. _____

15. _____

16. _____

17. _____

18. _____

19. _____

20. _____

21. _____

22. _____

23. _____

24. _____

25. _____

26. _____

27. _____

Name _____   Score _____

Solve.

The relationship between Celsius temperature and Fahrenheit temperature is given by the formula
$C = \dfrac{5}{9}(F - 32)$, **where** C **is the Celsius temperature and** F **is the Fahrenheit temperature.**

1. Find the Fahrenheit temperature when   2. Find the Fahrenheit temperature when   1. _____
    the Celsius temperature is 95°.   the Celsius temperature is –22°.

                                                                                                2. _____

Use the formula $T = U \cdot N + F$, **where** T **is the total cost,** U **is the unit cost,** N **is the number of units made, and** F **is the fixed cost.**

3. A computer table manufacturer's fixed   4. A blender manufacturer's fixed cost   3. _____
    cost per month are $9000. The unit cost   per month is $7000. The unit cost for
    for each table is $150. Find the number   each blender is $18. Find the number
    of tables made during a month in   of blenders made during a month in
    which the total cost was $99,000.   which the total cost was $79,000.
                                                                                                4. _____

Use the formula $M = S \cdot R + B$, **where** M **is the monthly earnings,** S **is the total sales,** R **is the commission rate, and** B **is the base monthly salary.**

5. A sales executive receives a base   6. A manager of a fast food store   5. _____
    monthly salary of $1000 plus a 6%   receives a base monthly salary of
    commission on total sales. Find the $780 plus a 3% commission on
    executive's monthly earning during a   total sales. Find the total sales during
    month in which the total sales were   a month in which the manager earned
    $42,000. $3180?   6. _____

Use the formula $V = V_0 + 32t$, **where** V **is the final velocity of a falling object,** V_0 **is the starting velocity of a falling object, and** t **is the time for the object to fall.**

7. Find the time required for a falling   8. Find the time required for an object   7. _____
    object to increase in velocity from   to reach a velocity of 729 ft/s when
    9 ft/s to 81 ft/s.   dropped from a helicopter. (The
                                                    starting velocity is 0 ft/s).
                                                                                                8. _____

Name   Score

Solve.

1. $2x + 7 = x + 2$ 2. $7x + 4 = 3x - 8$ 3. $3x + 5 = x - 11$

4. $8x + 7 = 3x - 8$ 5. $3x - 10 = x - 6$ 6. $7x - 4 = 8x - 3$

7. $6x - 9 = 2x + 15$ 8. $x - 5 = 3x - 9$ 9. $3x - 4 = 5 - 6x$

10. $2x + 9 = 7x - 6$ 11. $8 - 5x = 14 - 4x$ 12. $6x + 1 = 3x + 19$

13. $8 - 2x = 5 - x$ 14. $4x - 10 = 3x - 19$ 15. $11x - 8 = 3x - 16$

16. $6x - 7 = -3x - 20$ 17. $3x - 9 = -x + 15$ 18. $x + 15 = 4x - 15$

19. $7 - 2x = 9x + 7$ 20. $-6x + 3 = 3x - 15$ 21. $-1 - 6x = 7 - 2x$

22. $-5 + 8x = 7 + 7x$ 23. $5 - 3x = 4x - 9$ 24. $3x + 12 = -6x - 6$

1. _____
2. _____
3. _____
4. _____
5. _____
6. _____
7. _____
8. _____
9. _____
10. _____
11. _____
12. _____
13. _____
14. _____
15. _____
16. _____
17. _____
18. _____
19. _____
20. _____
21. _____
22. _____
23. _____
24. _____

Name _____   Score _____

Solve.

1. $-2+6(x+5)=-2$ **2.** $7x-2(x-3)=11$ **3.** $3+6(x+3)=12$

4. $7-2(x+1)=17$ **5.** $3x+2(x-4)=22$ **6.** $2x-3(x+2)=15$

7. $3x-4(x+1)=9$ **8.** $5x-3(x-2)=10$ **9.** $4(x-3)+7=7$

10. $2x+5(x-1)=2$ **11.** $7x-5(x+6)=18$ **12.** $4x-3(x+1)=7$

13. $3x+4(x-2)=6$ **14.** $6x-2(x+4)=16$ **15.** $4x-3(x+3)=-2$

16. $7x+2(x-1)=25$ **17.** $3x-4(x-2)=9$ **18.** $5x-4(x+2)=4$

19. $3x-3(x-5)=5(x+2)$ **20.** $x+3(x+2)=5(x+1)$ **21.** $4x-3(x-2)=2(x-1)$

22. $6x-2(x+1)=3(x+2)$ **23.** $7-(x+2)=2(x+4)$ **24.** $8x-6(x-2)=4(x+3)$

1. _____
2. _____
3. _____
4. _____
5. _____
6. _____
7. _____
8. _____
9. _____
10. _____
11. _____
12. _____
13. _____
14. _____
15. _____
16. _____
17. _____
18. _____
19. _____
20. _____
21. _____
22. _____
23. _____
24. _____

Name _____   Score _____

Translate into a mathematical expression.

1. 8 more than x

2. 3 less than c

3. the product of x and 5

4. y divided by c

5. two times the sum of m and n

6. the difference between m and n

7. x increased by the cube of x

8. v less than twice the square of v

9. the sum of x and one half of y

10. the product of a and one third of a

11. the difference between x and the square of x

12. the product of x and the sum of x and 3

13. the quotient of 1 less than x and x

14. x increased by the quotient of x and 5

15. y divided by the total of y and 1

16. the total of y and 1 divided by y

17. the sum of c and the product of 2 and c

18. m less than one sixth of m

19. b divided by the total of 3 and b

20. Four more than the product of x and y

21. the difference of x and the product of 3 and x

1. _____

2. _____

3. _____

4. _____

5. _____

6. _____

7. _____

8. _____

9. _____

10. _____

11. _____

12. _____

13. _____

14. _____

15. _____

16. _____

17. _____

18. _____

19. _____

20. _____

21. _____

Name

Score

Translate into a mathematical expression.

1.	8 more than a number	2.	6 less than a number	3.	6 less than a number

1. _____

2. _____

3. _____

4. the product of –3 and some number

5. the sum of one half of a number and the number

6. the sum of a number and the square of the number

4. _____

5. _____

6. _____

7. the product of a number and the sum of the number and 2

8. a number decreased by twice the number

9. the total of a number and the quotient of the number and 3

7. _____

8. _____

9. _____

10. the product of a number and one third of the number

11. the quotient of 4 more than a number and the number

12. the total of a number and seven times the square of the number

10. _____

11. _____

12. _____

13. the product of a number and the sum of the number and 1

14. 1 less than one fifth of some number

15. the cube of some number

13. _____

14. _____

15. _____

16. a number plus 11

17. two less than some number

18. three times some number

16. _____

17. _____

18. _____

19. a number divided by twelve

20. two thirds of a number

21. two increased by some number

19. _____

20. _____

21. _____

Name _____ Score _____

Translate into an equation and solve.

1. The product of four and a number is twenty-four. Find the number.

2. The quotient of a number and six is five. Find the number.

1. _____

2. _____

3. Nine more than a number is one. Find the number.

4. A number divided by twelve is three. Find the number.

3. _____

4. _____

5. Five times a number is twenty-four. Find the number.

6. Two-thirds of a number is eighteen. Find the number.

5. _____

6. _____

7. The total of eleven and a number is four. Find the number.

8. The sum of twice a number and five is thirteen. Find the number.

7. _____

8. _____

9. One fourth of a number and five is eight. Find the number.

10. Five less than four times a number is eleven. Find the number.

9. _____

10. _____

11. The total of a number divided by three and four is two. Find the number.

12. The sum of a number divided by eight and ten is two. Find the number.

11. _____

12. _____

13. The ratio of a number to seven is eleven. Find the number.

14. Four increased by two times a number is 40. Find the number.

13. _____

14. _____

15. Six more than the quotient of a number and four is equal to negative three. Find the number.

16. One decreased by the quotient of a number and five is two. Find the number.

15. _____

16. _____

Name   Score

Write and equation and solve.

1. A dental assistant paid $2640 in state income tax this year. This is $158 more than last year. Find the state income tax last year.

2. A video store is selling a VCR for $99. This is $20 more than the price at a catalog store. Find the price at the catalog store.

1. _____

2. _____

3. The value of a beach condo this year is $130,500. This is 16% higher than its price last year. Find its price last year.

4. During a sale, a television set is discounted $60. This is 15% off the regular price. Find the regular price.

3. _____

4. _____

5. A city's population has increased by 40,000 within the last four years. This represents a 10% increase. Find the city's population four years ago.

6. The selling price of a pair of water skis is $119.40. This price includes the store's cost for purchasing the skis plus a markup of 33%. Find the store's cost for the skis.

5. _____

6. _____

7. The monthly income for a manager of a mobile home dealership was $2200. This includes the manager base salary of $1200 plus a 1% commission on the total sales. Find the total sales for the month.

8. A laptop computer is bought for $2600. A down payment of $650 is made. The remainder of the cost is paid in 30 equal payments. Find the monthly payments.

7. _____

8. _____

9. A roofing contractor charges $100 plus $65 for each square of roofing material installed. How many squares of roofing material can be installed for $1140?

10. Each month an employee has $150 invested in a stock investment plan. This amounts to one tenth of the employee's monthly salary. Find the monthly salary.

9. _____

10. _____

CHAPTER 1

Objective 1.1A

1.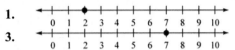

2.

3.

4.

5. >　**6.** >　**7.** <　**8.** <　**9.** >　**10.** <　**11.** <　**12.** >　**13.** <　**14.** >　**15.** >　**16.** <

Objective 1.1B

1. Eight hundred sixty-two　**2.** Three hundred eight　**3.** Six hundred fifty-four
4. Five thousand one hundred twenty-five　**5.** Nine thousand forty
6. Thirty-six thousand eight hundred forty-four　**7.** Three hundred eighty thousand seven hundred fifty-one
8. Eight hundred thousand one　**9.** Seven million six hundred forty thousand seven hundred twenty-three
10. 33　**11.** 274　**12.** 9527　**13.** 56,320　**14.** 460,303　**15.** 4,012,986　**16.** 1,000,0005　**17.** 8,001,050

Objective 1.1C

1. $200 + 50 + 6$　**2.** $4000 + 700 + 3$　**3.** $9000 + 200 + 30 + 3$　**4.** $20,000 + 3000 + 40$
5. $50,000 + 900 + 10 + 6$　**6.** $70,000 + 5000 + 40 + 9$　**7.** $90,000 + 9000 + 2$
8. $200,000 + 30,000 + 4000 + 700 + 80 + 2$　**9.** $500,000 + 400$　**10.** $700,000 + 80,000 + 7000$
11. $800,000 + 6000 + 8$　**12.** $900,000 + 20,000 + 10$　**13.** $4,000,000 + 200,000 + 70,000 + 1000 + 20$
14. $6,000,000 + 200 + 10 + 3$

Objective 1.1D

1. 750　**2.** 710　**3.** 400　**4.** 600　**5.** 1100　**6.** 7100　**7.** 4000　**8.** 10,000
9. 75,000　**10.** 69,000　**11.** 250,000　**12.** 840,000　**13.** 3,000,000　**14.** 8,000,000

Objective 1.2A

1. 866　**2.** 852　**3.** 2595　**4.** 18,340　**5.** 20,631　**6.** 19,630　**7.** 17,717　**8.** 21,434
9. 22,553　**10.** 231,792　**11.** 306,459　**12.** 267,879　**13.** 1439　**14.** 1271
15. 34,239　**16.** 73,369　**17.** 14,716　**18.** 16,140　**19.** 74,748　**20.** 34,430
21. 92,416　**22.** 8,962,349

Objective 1.2B

1. $81　**2.** $340　**3.** 3235 people　**4.** 239 people　**5.** $15,570　**6.** 889 toasters　**7.** $1554
8. 62,363 miles　**9.** $1790　**10.** $8,643,446

Objective 1.3A

1. 5　**2.** 3　**3.** 1　**4.** 15　**5.** 11　**6.** 61　**7.** 95　**8.** 400　**9.** 71　**10.** 561　**11.** 222
12. 303　**13.** 8413　**14.** 817　**15.** 2204　**16.** 1115　**17.** 1252　**18.** 2131　**19.** 21
20. 8　**21.** 821　**22.** 811　**23.** 7006　**24.** 421　**25.** 2111　**26.** 6151

Objective 1.3B

1. 44　**2.** 58　**3.** 59　**4.** 88　**5.** 54　**6.** 179　**7.** 3269　**8.** 4399　**9.** 966　**10.** 2430
11. 812　**12.** 3819　**13.** 3919　**14.** 26,699　**15.** 43,848　**16.** 19,027　**17.** 151,271　**18.** 353,874
19. 375　**20.** 637　**21.** 4676　**22.** 7481　**23.** 24,789　**24.** 56,741　**25.** 26,907　**26.** 15,582

Objective 1.3C

1. $23   **2.** $7724   **3.** 10,576 miles   **4.** 53,807 miles   **5.** $211   **6.** $650   **7.** $3220
8. $366   **9.** $385   **10.** 169,064 square miles

Objective 1.4A

1. 63   **2.** 0   **3.** 20   **4.** 48   **5.** 15   **6.** 36   **7.** 207   **8.** 168   **9.** 426   **10.** 245   **11.** 684
12. 152   **13.** 316   **14.** 5192   **15.** 1638   **16.** 4225   **17.** 3885   **18.** 2523
19. 7952   **20.** 28,326   **21.** 71,046   **22.** 26,172   **23.** 17,592   **24.** 18,620   **25.** 51,702
26. 363,930   **27.** 410,544

Objective 1.4B

1. 392   **2.** 1860   **3.** 3150   **4.** 649   **5.** 1755   **6.** 7968   **7.** 17,984   **8.** 18,315
9. 47,320   **10.** 60,776   **11.** 11,250   **12.** 22,743   **13.** 203,190   **14.** 427,118   **15.** 730,576
16. 183,732   **17.** 445,200   **18.** 105,248   **19.** 181,815   **20.** 601,644   **21.** 198,170   **22.** 1,871,773
23. 2,235,162   **24.** 3,014,525   **25.** 864,000   **26.** 1,154,160   **27.** 2,998,128

Objective 1.4C

1. 228 miles   **2.** 318 miles   **3.** 864 books   **4.** $9456   **5.** $3048   **6.** $584   **7.** 8508 hours
8. $630   **9.** 63,200 gallons   **10.** $7,999,680

Objective 1.5A

1. 2   **2.** 2   **3.** 1   **4.** 12   **5.** 7   **6.** 4   **7.** 19   **8.** 8   **9.** 11   **10.** 135   **11.** 125   **12.** 82
13. 49   **14.** 525   **15.** 456   **16.** 527   **17.** 399   **18.** 5561   **19.** 11,479
20. 5234   **21.** 7639

Objective 1.5B

1. 2 r 1   **2.** 4 r 1   **3.** 1 r 1   **4.** 4 r 5   **5.** 15 r 2   **6.** 12 r 1   **7.** 18 r 1
8. 6 r 6   **9.** 4 r 4   **10.** 173 r 1   **11.** 50 r 5   **12.** 148 r 2   **13.** 53 r 4   **14.** 392 r 2
15. 991 r 2   **16.** 692 r 6   **17.** 1478 r 1   **18.** 7446 r 4   **19.** 8217 r 1   **20.** 14,850 r 3   **21.** 9080 r 1

Objective 1.5C

1. 4 r 2   **2.** 1 r 37   **3.** 1 r 31   **4.** 5 r 9   **5.** 7   **6.** 12 r 22   **7.** 5 r 9
8. 128 r 26   **9.** 103 r 10   **10.** 144 r 9   **11.** 121   **12.** 80 r 18   **13.** 85 r 6   **14.** 74 r 29
15. 186 r 28   **16.** 61 r 32   **17.** 69 r 57   **18.** 591 r 20   **19.** 794 r 8   **20.** 83 r 110   **21.** 79

Objective 1.5D

1. 15,000 bushels   **2.** 564   **3.** $184,250   **4.** 160 people   **5.** $212   **6.** $39
7. $115   **8.** $184   **9.** $102,563   **10.** 256 packages

Objective 1.6A

1. 4^4 **2.** 8^6 **3.** $3^4 \cdot 4^2$ **4.** $5^4 \cdot 7^3$ **5.** $2 \cdot 6^7$ **6.** $6 \cdot 10^4$ **7.** $2^3 \cdot 3^4 \cdot 7^2$ **8.** $5 \cdot 6 \cdot 7^2 \cdot 8^3$
9. $4^2 \cdot 5^3 \cdot 6^3 \cdot 7$ **10.** $7^3 \cdot 15^2 \cdot 19^2$ **11.** 16   **12.** 27   **13.** 64   **14.** 3888
15. 2000   **16.** 25,088   **17.** 0   **18.** 320   **19.** 37,500   **20.** 102,900   **21.** 13,824
22. 38,690   **23.** 139,968   **24.** 0   **25.** 14,400

Objective 1.6B

1. 10 **2.** 11 **3.** 19 **4.** 0 **5.** 8 **6.** 5 **7.** 6 **8.** 11 **9.** 8 **10.** 10 **11.** 79 **12.** 0 **13.** 23 **14.** 0
15. 22 **16.** 16 **17.** 84 **18.** 7 **19.** 2 **20.** 38 **21.** 13 **22.** 8 **23.** 33 **24.** 4 **25.** 9 **26.** 5 **27.** 10

Objective 1.7A

1. 1, 2 **2.** 1, 2, 7, 14 **3.** 1, 3, 7, 21 **4.** 1, 3, 5, 15 **5.** 1, 23 **6.** 1, 2, 4, 5, 8, 10, 20, 40
7. 1, 2, 19, 38 **8.** 1, 2, 3, 4, 5, 6, 10, 12, 15, 20, 30, 60 **9.** 1, 2, 29, 58 **10.** 1, 2, 31, 62 **11.** 1, 3, 9, 27, 81
12. 1, 3, 17, 51 **13.** 1, 3, 9, 11, 33, 99 **14.** 1, 5, 17, 85 **15.** 1, 2, 5, 7, 10, 14, 35, 70
16. 1, 2, 4, 8, 11, 22, 44, 88 **17.** 1, 3, 7, 9, 21, 63 **18.** 1, 5, 7, 35 **19.** 1, 3, 5, 9, 15, 45
20. 1, 2, 3, 6, 13, 26, 39, 78 **21.** 1, 5, 11, 55 **22.** 1, 2, 57, 114 **23.** 1, 11, 121 **24.** 1, 3, 9, 13, 39, 117
25. 1, 2, 3, 5, 6, 10, 15, 25, 30 50, 75, 150 **26.** 1, 5, 7, 25, 35, 175 **27.** 1, 181

Objective 1.7B

1. $2 \cdot 2 \cdot 2$ **2.** $2 \cdot 3 \cdot 5$ **3.** $1 \cdot 53$ **4.** $2 \cdot 5$ **5.** $2 \cdot 2 \cdot 2 \cdot 2 \cdot 2$ **6.** $2 \cdot 2 \cdot 2 \cdot 2 \cdot 2 \cdot 2$ **7.** $1 \cdot 11$
8. $2 \cdot 2 \cdot 5$ **9.** $2 \cdot 41$ **10.** $5 \cdot 7$ **11.** $2 \cdot 2 \cdot 11$ **12.** $3 \cdot 23$ **13.** $2 \cdot 2 \cdot 2 \cdot 3 \cdot 3$
14. $2 \cdot 2 \cdot 2 \cdot 11$ **15.** $2 \cdot 47$ **16.** $2 \cdot 2 \cdot 3 \cdot 5$ **17.** $7 \cdot 11$ **18.** $2 \cdot 2 \cdot 5 \cdot 5$ **19.** $2 \cdot 2 \cdot 2 \cdot 13$ **20.** $2 \cdot 2 \cdot 2 \cdot 2 \cdot 7$
21. $2 \cdot 2 \cdot 31$ **22.** $2 \cdot 5 \cdot 13$ **23.** $5 \cdot 31$ **24.** $2 \cdot 2 \cdot 2 \cdot 5 \cdot 5$ **25.** $3 \cdot 3 \cdot 5 \cdot 7$ **26.** $2 \cdot 2 \cdot 5 \cdot 5 \cdot 5$ **27.** $2 \cdot 2 \cdot 5 \cdot 13$

CHAPTER 2

Objective 2.1A

1. 12 **2.** 21 **3.** 18 **4.** 40 **5.** 8 **6.** 36 **7.** 36 **8.** 30 **9.** 48 **10.** 75 **11.** 224 **12.** 36
13. 216 **14.** 252 **15.** 128 **16.** 63 **17.** 108 **18.** 231 **19.** 72
20. 200 **21.** 84 **22.** 154 **23.** 224 **24.** 80 **25.** 216 **26.** 36 **27.** 32

Objective 2.1B

1. 1 **2.** 3 **3.** 1 **4.** 2 **5.** 5 **6.** 5 **7.** 15 **8.** 4 **9.** 9 **10.** 7 **11.** 5 **12.** 10 **13.** 16
14. 13 **15.** 1 **16.** 2 **17.** 1 **18.** 3 **19.** 1 **20.** 5 **21.** 8 **22.** 4 **23.** 8 **24.** 9 **25.** 14 **26.** 17 **27.** 15

Objective 2.2A

1. $\frac{5}{8}$ **2.** $\frac{5}{7}$ **3.** $\frac{3}{5}$ **4.** $\frac{1}{4}$ **5.** $1\frac{2}{3}$ **6.** $1\frac{3}{4}$ **7.** $2\frac{4}{5}$ **8.** $2\frac{1}{2}$

9. $3\frac{1}{2}$ **10.** $3\frac{7}{8}$ **11.** $2\frac{3}{8}$ **12.** $2\frac{5}{8}$ **13.** $2\frac{1}{5}$ **14.** $3\frac{1}{3}$

Objective 2.2B

1. $3\frac{2}{3}$ **2.** 6 **3.** $1\frac{8}{9}$ **4.** $4\frac{1}{2}$ **5.** $2\frac{2}{3}$ **6.** $4\frac{3}{4}$ **7.** 3 **8.** $1\frac{5}{6}$

9. 1 **10.** 8 **11.** 14 **12.** 5 **13.** $\frac{11}{5}$ **14.** $\frac{23}{3}$ **15.** $\frac{43}{9}$ **16.** $\frac{23}{8}$

17. $\frac{37}{7}$ **18.** $\frac{33}{5}$ **19.** $\frac{43}{4}$ **20.** $\frac{97}{10}$ **21.** $\frac{77}{6}$ **22.** $\frac{118}{15}$ **23.** $\frac{34}{3}$

24. $\frac{131}{8}$

Objective 2.3A

1. 26 **2.** 15 **3.** 32 **4.** 5 **5.** 21 **6.** 18 **7.** 15 **8.** 36 **9.** 12 **10.** 32 **11.** 55 **12.** 35 **13.** 72
14. 54 **15.** 120 **16.** 18 **17.** 34 **18.** 100 **19.** 60 **20.** 68
21. 44 **22.** 96 **23.** 315 **24.** 35 **25.** 195 **26.** 322 **27.** 903

Objective 2.3B

1. $\frac{2}{3}$ **2.** $\frac{3}{5}$ **3.** $\frac{1}{8}$ **4.** $\frac{4}{7}$ **5.** $\frac{2}{3}$ **6.** $\frac{5}{8}$ **7.** $\frac{5}{6}$ **8.** $1\frac{1}{3}$ **9.** 0 **10.** $\frac{5}{8}$ **11.** $\frac{1}{2}$ **12.** $\frac{7}{18}$ **13.** $\frac{1}{4}$

14. $\frac{7}{12}$ **15.** 3 **16.** $\frac{13}{18}$ **17.** $\frac{8}{9}$ **18.** $\frac{1}{3}$ **19.** $1\frac{4}{13}$ **20.** $\frac{1}{7}$ **21.** $\frac{8}{17}$ **22.** $\frac{13}{30}$

23. $\frac{23}{50}$ **24.** $\frac{26}{75}$ **25.** $\frac{7}{10}$ **26.** $\frac{11}{14}$ **27.** 4

Objective 2.4A

1. $\frac{5}{6}$ **2.** $1\frac{1}{10}$ **3.** $\frac{10}{19}$ **4.** $\frac{6}{7}$ **5.** $\frac{7}{8}$ **6.** 1 **7.** 2 **8.** $\frac{2}{7}$ **9.** $1\frac{4}{5}$ **10.** $\frac{15}{17}$ **11.** $\frac{3}{4}$ **12.** 1

13. $2\frac{1}{3}$ **14.** $1\frac{7}{9}$ **15.** $1\frac{3}{11}$ **16.** $2\frac{1}{2}$ **17.** $\frac{11}{12}$ **18.** $2\frac{1}{3}$ **19.** $\frac{13}{15}$

20. $1\frac{1}{5}$ **21.** $4\frac{1}{4}$ **22.** $2\frac{1}{5}$ **23.** $1\frac{2}{7}$ **24.** $1\frac{3}{16}$ **25.** $2\frac{3}{13}$ **26.** $1\frac{15}{17}$

27. $1\frac{8}{9}$

Objective 2.4B

1. $\frac{11}{12}$ **2.** $\frac{37}{45}$ **3.** $1\frac{13}{24}$ **4.** $1\frac{7}{16}$ **5.** $1\frac{11}{18}$ **6.** $1\frac{5}{24}$ **7.** $1\frac{16}{21}$

8. $1\frac{1}{42}$ **9.** $1\frac{21}{40}$ **10.** $1\frac{1}{8}$ **11.** $1\frac{1}{12}$ **12.** $1\frac{3}{4}$ **13.** $\frac{11}{12}$ **14.** $1\frac{17}{30}$

15. $1\frac{20}{21}$ **16.** $1\frac{17}{36}$ **17.** $1\frac{23}{24}$ **18.** $2\frac{4}{315}$ **19.** $1\frac{9}{16}$ **20.** $2\frac{13}{90}$ **21.** $1\frac{4}{5}$

22. $1\frac{6}{7}$ **23.** $2\frac{5}{18}$ **24.** $2\frac{11}{28}$ **25.** $1\frac{13}{40}$ **26.** $\frac{59}{165}$ **27.** $2\frac{1}{3}$

Objective 2.4C

1. $6\frac{1}{9}$ **2.** $9\frac{1}{2}$ **3.** $13\frac{9}{28}$ **4.** $17\frac{7}{12}$ **5.** $11\frac{19}{28}$ **6.** $11\frac{8}{45}$ **7.** $12\frac{1}{6}$ **8.** $10\frac{7}{10}$

9. $11\frac{6}{35}$ **10.** $13\frac{5}{18}$ **11.** $10\frac{9}{20}$ **12.** $29\frac{15}{56}$ **13.** $30\frac{29}{30}$ **14.** $21\frac{17}{18}$ **15.** $8\frac{17}{56}$

16. $14\frac{49}{60}$ **17.** $45\frac{21}{22}$ **18.** $28\frac{1}{60}$ **19.** $15\frac{7}{12}$ **20.** $20\frac{13}{70}$ **21.** $23\frac{7}{36}$ **22.** $17\frac{17}{24}$

23. $12\frac{3}{4}$ **24.** $32\frac{9}{20}$ **25.** $33\frac{23}{24}$ **26.** $25\frac{19}{20}$ **27.** $18\frac{5}{7}$

Objective 2.4D

1. $3\frac{1}{8}$ inches **2.** $2\frac{1}{16}$ inches **3.** $3\frac{7}{8}$ inches **4.** $\$23\frac{1}{8}$ **5.** $4\frac{5}{16}$ inches **6.** $7\frac{1}{2}$ hours

7. $19\frac{3}{8}$ long and $14\frac{5}{8}$ inches wide **8.** $3\frac{1}{4}$ pounds **9.** $7\frac{3}{8}$ cups **10.** $\$204$

Objective 2.5A

1. $\frac{1}{6}$ 2. $\frac{5}{12}$ 3. $\frac{1}{3}$ 4. $\frac{8}{15}$ 5. $\frac{4}{5}$ 6. $\frac{1}{7}$ 7. $\frac{12}{25}$

8. $\frac{3}{10}$ 9. $\frac{3}{8}$ 10. $\frac{1}{2}$ 11. $\frac{6}{11}$ 12. $\frac{8}{23}$ 13. $\frac{3}{7}$ 14. $\frac{14}{27}$

15. $\frac{2}{13}$ 16. $\frac{3}{8}$ 17. $\frac{1}{3}$ 18. $\frac{9}{13}$ 19. $\frac{1}{6}$ 20. $\frac{8}{9}$ 21. $\frac{7}{10}$

22. $\frac{7}{10}$ 23. $\frac{5}{7}$ 24. $\frac{4}{35}$ 25. $\frac{8}{19}$ 26. $\frac{11}{29}$ 27. $\frac{4}{11}$

Objective 2.5B

1. $\frac{7}{20}$ 2. $\frac{1}{10}$ 3. $\frac{1}{7}$ 4. $\frac{22}{147}$ 5. $\frac{13}{32}$ 6. $\frac{32}{57}$ 7. $\frac{68}{135}$

8. $\frac{31}{80}$ 9. $\frac{1}{78}$ 10. $\frac{10}{21}$ 11. $\frac{3}{20}$ 12. $\frac{29}{90}$ 13. $\frac{17}{54}$ 14. $\frac{1}{12}$

15. $\frac{29}{60}$ 16. $\frac{31}{99}$ 17. $\frac{19}{175}$ 18. $\frac{25}{72}$ 19. $\frac{7}{20}$ 20. $\frac{9}{35}$ 21. $\frac{3}{10}$

22. $\frac{13}{30}$ 23. $\frac{1}{10}$ 24. $\frac{31}{42}$ 25. $\frac{11}{72}$ 26. $\frac{1}{78}$ 27. $\frac{7}{40}$

Objective 2.5C

1. $4\frac{4}{11}$ 2. $15\frac{1}{4}$ 3. $41\frac{1}{3}$ 4. $9\frac{15}{26}$ 5. $4\frac{1}{16}$ 6. $7\frac{3}{5}$ 7. $18\frac{3}{7}$

8. $21\frac{5}{7}$ 9. $3\frac{3}{5}$ 10. $29\frac{17}{18}$ 11. $32\frac{14}{135}$ 12. $23\frac{17}{35}$ 13. $24\frac{7}{48}$ 14. $35\frac{5}{12}$

15. $48\frac{45}{56}$ 16. $13\frac{29}{45}$ 17. $34\frac{1}{48}$ 18. $8\frac{21}{25}$ 19. $5\frac{7}{40}$ 20. $38\frac{67}{70}$ 21. $8\frac{35}{36}$

22. $9\frac{1}{6}$ 23. $2\frac{17}{30}$ 24. $126\frac{15}{56}$ 25. $75\frac{9}{10}$ 26. $53\frac{13}{120}$ 27. $17\frac{23}{60}$

Objective 2.5D

1. $\frac{7}{12}$ inch 2. $1\frac{7}{9}$ feet 3. $\frac{2}{5}$ 4. $\frac{7}{12}$ feet 5. $5\frac{7}{24}$ feet 6. $2\frac{3}{4}$ hours 7. $10\frac{5}{8}$ miles

8. $9\frac{1}{4}$ pounds 9. $\frac{11}{20}$ 10. $1\frac{7}{8}$ miles

Objective 2.6A

1. $\frac{8}{13}$ 2. $\frac{6}{11}$ 3. $\frac{4}{27}$ 4. $\frac{3}{16}$ 5. $\frac{35}{66}$ 6. $\frac{13}{54}$ 7. $\frac{11}{28}$

8. $\frac{25}{72}$ 9. $\frac{7}{8}$ 10. $\frac{49}{90}$ 11. $2\frac{7}{8}$ 12. $\frac{16}{35}$ 13. $\frac{13}{20}$ 14. $\frac{15}{56}$

15. 2 16. $10\frac{6}{17}$ 17. $1\frac{57}{119}$ 18. $\frac{3}{8}$ 19. $1\frac{1}{27}$ 20. $\frac{15}{68}$ 21. $\frac{3}{22}$

22. $\frac{15}{28}$ 23. $\frac{3}{10}$ 24. $\frac{21}{25}$ 25. 1 26. $\frac{1}{18}$ 27. $\frac{66}{91}$

Answers to Drill-and-Practice Pages

Objective 2.6B

1. $3\frac{1}{2}$ 2. $1\frac{3}{11}$ 3. $4\frac{2}{7}$ 4. $2\frac{1}{2}$ 5. 25 6. $\frac{13}{30}$ 7. 33

8. $1\frac{10}{13}$ 9. $9\frac{4}{5}$ 10. $1\frac{10}{21}$ 11. 0 12. $55\frac{1}{3}$ 13. $53\frac{9}{10}$ 14. 90

15. $67\frac{15}{28}$ 16. $59\frac{1}{2}$ 17. $38\frac{1}{2}$ 18. 36 19. $35\frac{15}{17}$ 20. $7\frac{5}{16}$ 21. $108\frac{1}{2}$

22. $28\frac{7}{11}$ 23. 33 24. 267 25. $124\frac{2}{3}$ 26. $7\frac{4}{5}$ 27. 60

Objective 2.6C

1. $174 2. 119 miles 3. $2\frac{3}{16}$ feet 4. $1408 5. $864 6. $11,010 7. 258 pages

8. $5\frac{11}{16}$ miles 9. $486 10. 752 miles

Objective 2.7A

1. $\frac{1}{6}$ 2. $1\frac{1}{3}$ 3. $\frac{3}{20}$ 4. $\frac{3}{10}$ 5. $\frac{17}{33}$ 6. $3\frac{2}{3}$ 7. $\frac{1}{2}$

8. $\frac{1}{2}$ 9. $\frac{5}{7}$ 10. $3\frac{3}{4}$ 11. $\frac{2}{3}$ 12. $1\frac{3}{11}$ 13. 0 14. $1\frac{3}{8}$

15. $\frac{8}{35}$ 16. $5\frac{1}{4}$ 17. $\frac{2}{5}$ 18. $1\frac{5}{9}$ 19. $2\frac{5}{11}$ 20. $\frac{2}{15}$ 21. $\frac{1}{2}$

22. $\frac{19}{36}$ 23. 1 24. $1\frac{1}{5}$ 25. $\frac{4}{9}$ 26. 16 27. $\frac{2}{3}$

Objective 2.7B

1. $\frac{1}{7}$ 2. $9\frac{1}{2}$ 3. 90 4. $1\frac{1}{2}$ 5. $\frac{16}{55}$ 6. $\frac{2}{5}$ 7. $1\frac{17}{21}$

8. $1\frac{1}{4}$ 9. $1\frac{17}{40}$ 10. $\frac{26}{29}$ 11. 10 12. $\frac{1}{14}$ 13. $13\frac{7}{11}$ 14. $1\frac{1}{4}$

15. 15 16. $\frac{2}{5}$ 17. $\frac{1}{23}$ 18. $\frac{3}{13}$ 19. 2 20. $2\frac{15}{26}$ 21. $3\frac{1}{12}$

22. $\frac{5}{144}$ 23. $\frac{8}{29}$ 24. $2\frac{10}{29}$ 25. $1\frac{1}{11}$ 26. $28\frac{1}{2}$ 27. $1\frac{16}{21}$

Objective 2.7C

1. $624 2. 44 miles per hour 3. 20 miles 4. 48 questions 5. 66,000 registered voters

6. $12 7. 12 dolls 8. $48,000 9. $1\frac{1}{4}$ feet 10. 123 students

Objective 2.8A

1. < 2. > 3. > 4. < 5. < 6. > 7. > 8. > 9. < 10. < 11. < 12. > 13. > 14. <
15. < 16. < 17. > 18. < 19. < 20. > 21. < 22. > 23. < 24. < 25. > 26. < 27. >

Objective 2.8B

1. $\dfrac{25}{121}$ 2. $\dfrac{9}{49}$ 3. $\dfrac{25}{64}$ 4. $\dfrac{9}{35}$ 5. $\dfrac{20}{147}$ 6. $\dfrac{1}{100}$ 7. $\dfrac{1}{7}$

8. $\dfrac{1}{9}$ 9. $\dfrac{1}{128}$ 10. $\dfrac{1}{99}$ 11. $\dfrac{3}{32}$ 12. $\dfrac{32}{95}$ 13. $\dfrac{1}{15}$ 14. $\dfrac{9}{128}$

15. $\dfrac{1}{10}$ 16. $\dfrac{1}{16}$ 17. $\dfrac{1}{51}$ 18. $\dfrac{1}{7}$ 19. $\dfrac{1}{27}$ 20. $\dfrac{7}{10}$ 21. $\dfrac{1}{15}$

22. $2\dfrac{4}{7}$ 23. $\dfrac{2}{135}$ 24. $\dfrac{7}{54}$ 25. $\dfrac{3}{128}$ 26. $\dfrac{4}{77}$ 27. $\dfrac{1}{169}$

Objective 2.8C

1. $\dfrac{43}{84}$ 2. $\dfrac{41}{45}$ 3. $\dfrac{7}{8}$ 4. $1\dfrac{89}{105}$ 5. $\dfrac{7}{8}$ 6. $\dfrac{11}{16}$ 7. $\dfrac{103}{252}$

8. $\dfrac{109}{270}$ 9. $\dfrac{4}{9}$ 10. $1\dfrac{19}{22}$ 11. $\dfrac{25}{36}$ 12. $\dfrac{2}{5}$ 13. 0 14. $1\dfrac{3}{98}$

15. $\dfrac{2}{3}$ 16. $1\dfrac{2}{23}$ 17. $2\dfrac{7}{8}$ 18. $\dfrac{1}{36}$ 19. 1 20. $\dfrac{5}{18}$ 21. $\dfrac{1}{3}$

22. $\dfrac{5}{21}$ 23. $\dfrac{9}{88}$ 24. $1\dfrac{19}{90}$ 25. $\dfrac{11}{36}$ 26. $4\dfrac{1}{3}$ 27. $2\dfrac{1}{8}$

CHAPTER 3

Objective 3.1A

1. Thirty-nine hundredths   2. Eighty-one hundredths   3. Two and seven thousandths
4. Five and sixty-one thousandths   5. Fifteen and four tenths   6. Eighty-six ten-thousandths
7. Twenty-six and three hundred seventy-nine thousandths
8. Five hundred fourteen and three thousand one hundred eighteen ten-thousandths
9. One thousand seventy-eight and two hundred-thousandths   10. 0.834   11. 0.000052   12. 6.0101
13. 87.906   14. 462.035   15. 6014.1008   16. 25.07293   17. 91.0017

Objective 3.1B

1. 0.1   2. 9.1   3. 26.3   4. 96.5   5. 65.34   6. 13.01   7. 517.68
8. 792.25   9. 2.092   10. 6.280   11. 79.463   12. 51.004   13. 0.0420   14. 0.0036
15. 4.3763   16. 16.1119   17. 0.24967   18. 0.00912   19. 7.88010   20. 11.73241   21. 1
22. 4   23. 71   24. 0.004590   25. 0.100864   26. 2.111006

Objective 3.2A

1. 205.2844   2. 51.1918   3. 120.1664   4. 89.5197   5. 69.5793   6. 24.908   7. 61.5488
8. 9.3676   9. 277.9922   10. 113.069   11. 1.29   12. 1.55   13. 11.015   14. 18.91
15. 15.239   16. 39.107   17. 53.8362   18. 106.8338   19. 93.3431   20. 105.556   21. 57.992
22. 84.084   23. 160.351   24. 50.5418   25. 15.6153

Objective 3.2B

1. $2695.07   2. $52.58   3. 7.45 feet   4. 3.95 feet   5. 36.3 miles   6. 2651.8 miles   7. $4805.96
8. $1889.91   9. $120.35   10. $22,281.20

Answers to Drill-and-Practice Pages

Objective 3.3A

1. 32.377
2. 5.421
3. 136.8126
4. 593.587
5. 2.3191
6. 23.126
7. 62.446
8. 2.756
9. 6.8963
10. 0.062
11. 0.597
12. 3.091
13. 22.402
14. 0.1607
15. 1.808
16. 135.184
17. 361.688
18. 348.742
19. 37.0785
20. 18.2864
21. 181.186
22. 393.2374
23. 633.4404
24. 4.0159
25. 34.74909
26. 6.60157
27. 42.06339

Objective 3.3B

1. $3.17
2. 1.579 inches
3. 0.7 pounds
4. 55.38 seconds
5. 25°C
6. $824.42
7. $897.27
8. $24.47
9. $2720.69
10. $34,547.79

Objective 3.4A

1. 0.35
2. 1.92
3. 50.4
4. 2.28
5. 0.168
6. 22.95
7. 3.552
8. 0.0789
9. 0.04664
10. 0.2747
11. 10.58
12. 0.07062
13. 0.04712
14. 3.45285
15. 0.019154
16. 4.736
17. 0.456
18. 1.716
19. 82.1
20. 3.5
21. 6823.5
22. 68.5
23. 3.5
24. 34,000
25. 15.0788
26. 19.6935
27. 0.02142

Objective 3.4B

1. 37.5 inches
2. 113 miles
3. $3.41
4. $13.60
5. $6996
6. $515.10
7. $2744
8. $965.40
9. $460,275
10. $245,880

Objective 3.5A

1. 0.94
2. 3.2
3. 50
4. 86.5
5. 1.303
6. 0.31
7. 2.8
8. 470
9. 9.3
10. 7.7
11. 0.9
12. 29.4
13. 0.278
14. 19.51
15. 0.69
16. 0.080
17. 0.831
18. 0.008
19. 1
20. 16
21. 70
22. 0.723
23. 0.49875
24. 0.0037615
25. 24.8
26. 3.15
27. 0.626

Objective 3.5B

1. $9.90
2. $39.50
3. $107.06
4. 836 gallons
5. 23 hairdryers
6. 6.2 minutes
7. $144.39
8. $130.46
9. $3.25
10. 2.3 feet

Objective 3.6A

1. 0.714
2. 0.067
3. 0.417
4. 0.889
5. 0.214
6. 0.545
7. 2.588
8. 0.438
9. 5.667
10. 0.643
11. 0.857
12. 1.25
13. 8.136
14. 15.5
15. 0.53
16. 4.375
17. 41.3
18. 1.087
19. 6.333
20. 0.556
21. 3.545
22. 27.111
23. 6.571
24. 0.013
25. 0.944
26. 6.556
27. 10.571

Objective 3.6B

1. $\frac{7}{10}$
2. $\frac{9}{10}$
3. $\frac{23}{50}$
4. $\frac{37}{50}$
5. $\frac{3}{8}$
6. $\frac{41}{200}$
7. $2\frac{11}{20}$
8. $6\frac{3}{4}$
9. $18\frac{2}{5}$
10. $12\frac{3}{10}$
11. $9\frac{1}{5}$
12. $14\frac{1}{2}$
13. $4\frac{69}{500}$
14. $6\frac{8}{125}$
15. $3\frac{7}{20}$
16. $9\frac{93}{100}$
17. $\frac{29}{175}$
18. $\frac{14}{15}$
19. $\frac{1}{9}$
20. $4\frac{81}{100}$
21. $\frac{11}{200}$
22. $\frac{3}{200}$
23. $23\frac{31}{50}$
24. $\frac{11}{25}$
25. $\frac{5}{6}$
26. $\frac{151}{600}$
27. $\frac{7}{9}$

Objective 3.6C

1. < 2. < 3. > 4. > 5. > 6. < 7. < 8. < 9. > 10. < 11. < 12. < 13. > 14. <
15. > 16. < 17. < 18. > 19. < 20. > 21. > 22. > 23. < 24. < 25. < 26. > 27. <

CHAPTER 4

Objective 4.1A

1. $\frac{3}{7}$, 3:7, 3 to 7
2. $\frac{3}{8}$, 3:8, 3 to 8
3. $\frac{3}{5}$, 3:5, 3 to 5
4. $\frac{3}{4}$, 3:4, 3 to 4
5. $\frac{1}{7}$, 1:7, 1 to 7
6. $\frac{3}{7}$, 3:7, 3 to 7
7. $\frac{5}{1}$, 5:1, 5 to 1
8. $\frac{23}{14}$, 23:14, 23 to 14
9. $\frac{1}{1}$, 1:1, 1 to 1
10. $\frac{3}{2}$, 3:2, 3 to 2
11. $\frac{7}{4}$, 7:4, 7 to 4
12. $\frac{1}{3}$, 1:3, 1 to 3
13. $\frac{12}{11}$, 12:11, 12 to 11
14. $\frac{1}{5}$; 1:5, 1 to 5
15. $\frac{7}{8}$, 7:8, 7 to 8
16. $\frac{10}{9}$, 10:9, 10 to 9
17. $\frac{3}{4}$, 3:4, 3 to 4
18. $\frac{5}{11}$, 5:11, 5 to 11
19. $\frac{7}{6}$, 7:6, 7 to 6
20. $\frac{1}{6}$, 1:6, 1 to 6
21. $\frac{1}{2}$, 1:2, 1 to 2
22. $\frac{8}{5}$, 8:5, 8 to 5
23. $\frac{9}{4}$, 9:4, 9 to 4
24. $\frac{1}{1}$, 1:1, 1 to 1
25. $\frac{9}{10}$, 9:10, 9 to 10
26. $\frac{5}{2}$, 5:2, 5 to 2

Objective 4.1B

1. $\frac{1}{4}$
2. $\frac{11}{16}$
3. $\frac{18}{7}$
4. $\frac{4}{9}$
5. $\frac{3}{5}$
6. $\frac{5}{8}$
7. $\frac{3}{4}$
8. $\frac{23}{27}$
9. $\frac{6}{29}$
10. $\frac{3}{10}$

Objective 4.2A

1. $\frac{53 \text{ miles}}{2 \text{ hours}}$
2. $\frac{91 \text{ miles}}{3 \text{ gallons}}$
3. $\frac{26 \text{ feet}}{3 \text{ seconds}}$
4. $\frac{\$62}{3 \text{ toasters}}$
5. $\frac{\$303}{20 \text{ hours}}$
6. $\frac{\$3}{1 \text{ pound}}$
7. $\frac{\$501}{25 \text{ shares}}$
8. $\frac{1 \text{ tablet}}{6 \text{ hours}}$
9. $\frac{121 \text{ words}}{2 \text{ minutes}}$
10. $\frac{\$1525}{1 \text{ month}}$
11. $\frac{49 \text{ miles}}{1 \text{ hour}}$
12. $\frac{689 \text{ words}}{3 \text{ pages}}$
13. $\frac{\$13}{2 \text{ boards}}$
14. $\frac{3 \text{ clams}}{1 \text{ person}}$
15. $\frac{\$416}{1 \text{ week}}$
16. $\frac{8 \text{ place settings}}{1 \text{ table}}$
17. $\frac{41 \text{ pounds}}{3 \text{ square inches}}$
18. $\frac{\$7}{1 \text{ foot}}$
19. $\frac{\$1456}{1 \text{ department}}$
20. $\frac{217 \text{ seats}}{2 \text{ lecture halls}}$
21. $\frac{67 \text{ miles}}{2 \text{ gallons of gas}}$
22. $\frac{95 \text{ calls}}{2 \text{ hours}}$
23. $\frac{15 \text{ cups}}{1 \text{ urn}}$
24. $\frac{13 \text{ houses}}{51 \text{ acres}}$
25. $\frac{227 \text{ words}}{2 \text{ pages}}$
26. $\frac{\$13}{1 \text{ pound}}$

Objective 4.2B

1. $2.50/foot 2. 19 miles/gallon 3. 16.75 pounds/square inch 4. $24,000/partner 5. 8.4 gallons/minute
6. 49.8 miles/hour 7. 22.32 feet/second 8. $0.90/pound 9. 155 miles/day 10. 68 heartbeats/minute
11. $1500/month 12. 64 words/minute 13. $10.24/hour 14. $0.97/plant 15. 52.3 miles/hour
16. 7.3 pounds/square inch 17. $3.48/pound 18. 48 words/minute 19. 57 gallons/minute
20. 29.5 miles/gallon 21. $1250/partner 22. $6.72/hour 23. 72 heartbeats/minute 24. 126.9 miles/day
25. $1175/month 26. 12.3 feet/second

Objective 4.2C

1. $40.50 **2.** $2.59 **3.** 124 calls **4.** 57 words **5.** $0.67 **6.** $1.98 **7.** $83.57
8. $0.52 **9.** $1.80 **10.** $1.23

Objective 4.3A

1. True **2.** True **3.** True **4.** Not true **5.** True **6.** Not true **7.** Not true
8. True **9.** Not true **10.** True **11.** Not true **12.** Not true **13.** Not true **14.** True
15. Not true **16.** True **17.** Not true **18.** True **19.** True **20.** Not true **21.** Not true
22. True **23.** True **24.** Not true **25.** True **26.** Not true

Objective 4.3B

1. 6 **2.** 5 **3.** 12 **4.** 28 **5.** 24 **6.** 16.67 **7.** 24 **8.** 108 **9.** 10 **10.** 33.6 **11.** 6
12. 24.75 **13.** 24 **14.** 4.09 **15.** 6 **16.** 17.5 **17.** 7.5 **18.** 4.5 **19.** 47.5 **20.** 65.33
21. 17.5 **22.** 2.14 **23.** 1.2 **24.** 30 **25.** 27.35 **26.** 8.42 **27.** 22.92

Objective 4.3C

1. $90.40 **2.** 10.5 teaspoons **3.** $31.05 **4.** 34 feet **5.** $1036 **6.** $113.70
7. 2259 transistors **8.** $9.73 **9.** 10,380 people **10.** 434 gallons

CHAPTER 5

Objective 5.1A

1. $\frac{39}{100}$, 0.39 **2.** $\frac{16}{25}$, 0.64 **3.** $1\frac{1}{4}$, 1.25 **4.** $\frac{13}{50}$, 0.26 **5.** $\frac{17}{20}$, 0.80 **6.** $\frac{1}{5}$, 0.20 **7.** $4\frac{1}{4}$, 4.50

8. $\frac{19}{100}$, 0.19 **9.** $\frac{11}{20}$, 0.55 **10.** $\frac{71}{900}$ **11.** $\frac{23}{300}$ **12.** $\frac{129}{500}$ **13.** $\frac{129}{200}$ **14.** $\frac{13}{30}$

15. $\frac{399}{400}$ **16.** 0.675 **17.** 0.3407 **18.** 0.579 **19.** 0.40 **20.** 0.1389 **21.** 0.0201

Objective 5.1B

1. 32% **2.** 96% **3.** 4% **4.** 197% **5.** 214% **6.** 0.9% **7.** 68%
8. 12% **9.** 10.7% **10.** 41.7% **11.** 188.9% **12.** 57.1% **13.** 15.2% **14.** 60%

15. 183.3% **16.** $45\frac{5}{11}$% **17.** $22\frac{2}{9}$% **18.** $114\frac{2}{7}$% **19.** $37\frac{1}{2}$% **20.** $6\frac{2}{3}$% **21.** $58\frac{1}{3}$%

Objective 5.2A

1. 3.6 **2.** 15 **3.** 18.2 **4.** 47.7 **5.** 27 **6.** 19.25 **7.** 88.075
8. 12.688 **9.** 112 **10.** 0.05 **11.** 45 **12.** 0.2 **13.** 147 **14.** 13.2
15. 64.8 **16.** 5.25 **17.** 9.48 **18.** 11 **19.** 0.3 **20.** 36 **21.** 192.5
22. 38.75 **23.** 197 **24.** 60 **25.** 345.44 **26.** 84.15

Objective 5.2B

1. $7700 **2.** 400 employees **3.** $12.95 **4.** 2185 homes **5.** 486 plants **6.** 16.2 gallons
7. 2495 screws **8.** $19.98 **9.** $27,560 **10.** $188,000

Objective 5.3A

1. 31.25%   2. $16\frac{2}{3}$%   3. 80%   4. 60%   5. 20%   6. 45%   7. 300%
8. 250%   9. 15%   10. 36%   11. 4.5%   12. 4%   13. 75%   14. 10%
15. 30%   16. 5%   17. 500%   18. 11.25%   19. 0.5%   20. 5.5%   21. 30.5%
22. $33\frac{1}{3}$%   23. $66\frac{2}{3}$%   24. 20%   25. 9.5%   26. 150%

Objective 5.3B

1. 12% 2. 12% 3. 6%   4. 230%   5. 20% 6. 3%   7. 25% 8. 80% 9. 120%   10. 12.5%

Objective 5.4A

1. 185   2. 400   3. 50   4. 60   5. 100   6. 70   7. 123
8. 184   9. 5000   10. 800   11. 570   12. 16   13. 1100   14. 350
15. 45   16. 450   17. 21   18. 200   19. 890   20. 1700   21. 88.5
22. 57   23. 24   24. 258   25. 62   26. 78.25

Objective 5.4B

1. $12,500   2. 380 business establishments   3. 56 questions   4. 2700 books   5. 24 calls   6. $2.25
7. $800,000   8. 3 spaces   9. 790,000 DVDs   10. $7,500,000

Objective 5.5A

1. 289   2. 60   3. 30%   4. 35%   5. 60   6. 200   7. 50%
8. 25%   9. 510   10. 800   11. 37%   12. 450%   13. 768   14. 819
15. 60   16. 150   17. 40%   18. 52%   19. 5%   20. 12.5%   21. 350%
22. 400%   23. 16,500   24. 2500   25. 140   26. 7.25%

Objective 5.5B

1. 75%   2. $12\frac{1}{2}$%   3. $2.80   4. $75,600   5. $144   6. 97.5%   7. $8700
8. 7 errors   9. $10,500   10. 20%

CHAPTER 6

Objective 6.1A

1. $0.145 per ounce   2. $0.129 per ounce   3. $0.034 per ounce   4. $0.028 per ounce
5. $0.315 per ounce   6. $0.094 per ounce   7. $0.039 per ounce   8. $0.191 per ounce
9. $0.037 per ounce   10. $0.161 per ounce   11. $0.078 per ounce   12. $0.599 each   13. $0.297 each
14. $0.199 per ounce   15. 0.099 each   16. $0.423 per ounce   17. $0.034 per ounce
18. $0.258 per pound   19. $0.059 per ounce   20. $0.054 each   21. $0.055 per ounce   22. $0.042 each
23. $0.052 per ounce   24. $0.897 per pound

Objective 6.1B

1. 15 ounces for $0.94   2. 24 ounces for $0.94   3. 12 ounces for $1.30   4. 175 for $0.79   5. 50 for $1.89
6. 10 ounces for $0.74   7. 8 ounces for $0.89   8. 18 ounces for $1.39   9. 64 ounces for $1.35   10. 4 for $1.99
11. 9 for $1.27   12. $2.79 for 32 ounces   13. 16 ounces for $2.49   14. 2 pounds for $0.35   15. 8 ounces for $0.99
16. 10 pounds for $2.67   17. 18 ounces for $0.54   18. 6 ounces for $0.39   19. 50 for $1.09   20. $0.39 for 6.5 ounces
21. 9 ounces for $0.50   22. 119 sheets for $0.79   23. 12 ounces for $1.27   24. 12 ounces for $1.28

Answers to Drill-and-Practice Pages

Objective 6.1C

1. $7.16   **2.** $27.60   **3.** $7.96   **4.** $1.90   **5.** $1.17   **6.** $2.97   **7.** $0.66
8. $11.49   **9.** $1.25   **10.** $7.08   **11.** $10.60   **12.** $1.34   **13.** $10.04   **14.** $10.04
15. $12.50   **16.** $25.00

Objective 6.2A

1. 25%   **2.** $8\frac{1}{3}$%   **3.** $33\frac{1}{3}$%   **4.** 10%   **5.** 150 fans   **6.** 230 billboards

7a. $13.50   **7b.** $238.50   **8a.** $2560   **8b.** $34,560   **9a.** 50 spaces   **9b.** 5%
10a. 300 meters   **10b.** 4300 meters   **11.** 12.5%   **12.** 15%

Objective 6.2B

1. $7.80   **2.** $0.34   **3.** $10.88   **4.** 60%   **5a.** $13.60   **5b.** $47.60   **6a.** $19.80
6b. $64.80   **7a.** $0.60   **7b.** $1.69   **8a.** $9.10   **8b.** $35.10   **9.** $64.86   **10.** $44.64

Objective 6.2C

1. 15%   **2.** 30%   **3.** 12%   **4.** 15%   **5.** 81 employees   **6.** $375
7a. 6 minutes   **7b.** 37.5%   **8a.** 49 orders   **8b.** 35%   **9a.** $17,100   **9b.** $267,900   **10a.** $63
10b. $357   **11.** 24%   **12.** 5%

Objective 6.2D

1. 36%   **2.** 15%   **3.** $30   **4.** $75   **5.** 20%   **6.** $4.80   **7a.** $0.60
7b. $1.80   **8a.** $9.90   **8b.** $45.10   **9a.** $4.20   **9b.** 12%   **10a.** $120   **10b.** 20%
11. $138   **12.** $39

Objective 6.3A

1. $1800   **2.** $8960   **3.** $99,200   **4.** $14,790   **5.** $6225   **6.** $5.40   **7a.** $714
7b. $117.25   **8a.** $23,400   **8b.** $1841.67   **9a.** $56,250   **9b.** $2187.50   **10a.** $3608   **10b.** $246

Objective 6.3B

1. $264.64   **2.** $84.42   **3.** $375.43   **4.** $161.86   **5.** $166.03   **6.** $6.74   **7.** $8.57
8. $6.69

Objective 6.3C

1. $3864.07   **2.** $1693.34   **3.** $24,488.64   **4.** $425,635.60   **5.** $44,578.50   **6.** $17,287.76   **7a.** $23,566.40
7b. $19,566.40   **8a.** $124,840,80   **9a.** $36,387.16   **9b.** $1826.22   **10a.** $65,544.80   **10b.** Yes

Objective 6.4A

1. $215,000   **2.** $180,000   **3.** $18,075   **4.** $12,000   **5.** $31,500   **6.** $36,000   **7.** $2000
8. $5400   **9a.** $30,000   **9b.** $120,000   **10a.** $8800   **10b.** $79,200

Objective 6.4B

1. $973.88   **2.** $2875.60   **3.** Yes   **4.** No   **5.** $63.75   **6.** $56.67   **7a.** $1140.54
7b. $900   **8a.** $2086.88   **8b.** $1800   **9.** $1401.40   **10.** $1560.78

Objective 6.5A

1. $1020   **2.** No   **3.** $688.50   **4.** $442   **5.** $151.80   **6.** $201   **7a.** $286.60
7b. $2036.50   **8a.** $350   **8b.** $560   **9a.** $4800   **9b.** $19,200   **10.** $8925

Objective 6.5B

1. $189.85   **2.** $250.47   **3.** $3920   **4.** $208   **5.** $0.14   **6.** $0.11   **7.** $3530
8. $74.80   **9a.** $5000   **9b.** $173.33   **10a.** $9000   **10b.** $255.00   **11.** $267.40   **12.** $190.80

Objective 6.6A

1. $236.40   **2.** $288   **3.** $3650   **4.** $2125   **5.** $48.50   **6.** $78   **7.** $451
8. $1800   **9.** $450   **10.** $80   **11a.** $29.20   **11b.** $350.40   **12a.** $320,000   **12b.** $38,400

Objective 6.7A

1. $444.95   **2.** $568.36   **3.** $3153.42   **4.** $2344.70   **5.** $567.42   **6.** $232.03   **7.** Yes
8. No   **9.** Yes   **10.** No

Objective 6.7B

1. $495.06   **2.** $223.08   **3.** $325.34   **4.** $790.72   **5.** $1028.85   **6.** $721.72   **7.** $1197.44
8. $707.70   **9.** $1172.79   **10.** $1163.74

CHAPTER 7

Objective 7.1A

1. 1800 iPods   **2.** 550 iPods   **3.** 25%   **4.** $\frac{2}{3}$ **5.** 200 students   **6.** 125 students   **7.** 75 students   **8.** $\frac{5}{3}$

Objective 7.1B

1. $2280   **2.** $320   **3.** $1400   **4.** $\frac{12}{23}$ **5.** $\frac{2}{5}$ **6.** $\frac{1}{5}$ **7.** $\frac{7}{20}$ **8.** $\frac{1}{3}$

Objective 7.2A

1. $50,000   **2.** $55,000   **3.** $65,000   **4.** $40,000   **5.** 300 TVs   **6.** August   **7.** 100   **8.** 500 TVs

Objective 7.2B

1. $900,000   **2.** $1,200,000   **3.** September   **4.** December   **5.** $12,000,000   **6.** $5,000,000   **7.** $3,000,000
8. $22,000,000

Objective 7.3A

1. 20 cars   **2.** 5 cars   **3.** 50 cars   **4.** $\frac{1}{1}$ **5.** 25 employees   **6.** $\frac{1}{4}$
7. 60 employees   **8.** 50 employees

Objective 7.3B

1. 25 families   **2.** $\frac{5}{21}$ **3.** 30 families   **4.** $\frac{4}{7}$ **5.** 30 homes   **6.** $\frac{1}{5}$ **7.** 50 homes   **8.** 70 homes

Objective 7.4A

1. $16.32 **2.** 88 **3.** $273.20 **4.** 232 pizzas **5.** $36.75 **6.** 103 mi **7.** $8.38
8. 22 **9.** no mode **10.** 93

Objective 7.4B

1. 24 years **2.** 46 years **3.** 26 years **4.** 36 years **5.** 29 years **6.** 22 years **7.** 10 years
8. 75 **9.** 150 **10.** 75 **11.** 75% **12.** 0%

Objective 7.5A

1. $\frac{1}{12}$ **2.** $\frac{1}{9}$ **3.** 1 **4.** $\frac{3}{8}$ **5.** $\frac{4}{11}$ **6.** $\frac{2}{11}$

7. Drawing a diamond **8.** $\frac{2}{13}$ **9.** $\frac{1}{3}$ **10.** $\frac{1}{3}$

CHAPTER 8

Objective 8.1A

1. 60 in. **2.** 102 in. **3.** 112 in. **4.** 152 in. **5.** 5 ft **6.** $4\frac{1}{2}$ ft **7.** 6 ft

8. $5\frac{5}{6}$ ft **9.** 10 ft **10.** 14 ft **11.** 10 yd **12.** 6 yd **13.** 5 yd **14.** 198 in.

15. 2 yd **16.** $3\frac{1}{3}$ yd **17.** $2\frac{2}{3}$ yd **18.** 15,840 ft **19.** 23,760 ft **20.** 26,400 ft **21.** 12,320 ft

22. $11\frac{2}{3}$ ft **23.** 90 in. **24.** 81 in. **25.** 66 in. **26.** 2 mi **27.** $1\frac{1}{2}$ mi

Objective 8.1B

1. 1066 yd 2 ft **2.** 1 mi 1720 ft **3.** 13 ft 4 in. **4.** 1 mi 2720 ft **5.** 666 yd 2 ft **6.** 11 ft 8 in. **7.** 19 ft 11 in.
8. 3 ft 7 in. **9.** 35 ft **10.** 32 ft **11.** 42 ft **12.** 100 ft **13.** 1 ft 7 in. **14.** $8\frac{3}{4}$ ft

15. $16\frac{1}{12}$ ft **16.** $19\frac{1}{3}$ ft **17.** $1\frac{1}{2}$ ft **18.** $5\frac{1}{4}$ ft **19.** $8\frac{1}{8}$ yd **20.** 6 mi 720 ft

Objective 8.1C

1. $5\frac{1}{2}$ in. **2.** $1\frac{1}{8}$ ft **3.** 3 ft 2 in. **4.** $4\frac{1}{4}$ ft **5.** 126 ft **6.** 336 in. **7.** 8 ft 10 in.
8. 22.5 ft **9.** 74 ft **10.** $240.33

Objective 8.2A

1. 48 oz **2.** 2 lb **3.** 10,000 lb **4.** 8500 lb **5.** 4 tons **6.** $4\frac{3}{5}$ tons **7.** 1200 lb

8. 1250 lb **9.** 12,400 lb **10.** 224 oz **11.** $3\frac{1}{5}$ tons **12.** $1\frac{4}{5}$ tons **13.** $6\frac{1}{4}$ lb **14.** $5\frac{5}{8}$ lb

15. $18\frac{3}{4}$ lb **16.** 6200 lb **17.** 10,800 lb **18.** $2\frac{1}{4}$ tons **19.** 5200 lb **20.** 12 lb **21.** 156 oz

22. $10\frac{1}{2}$ lb **23.** $3\frac{7}{8}$ lb **24.** 5 lb **25.** 124 oz **26.** 70 oz **27.** 800 lb

Objective 8.2B

1. 3 tons 1000 lb **2.** 4 lb 12 oz **3.** 5 lb 10 oz **4.** 6 lb 4 oz **5.** 8 lb 12 oz **6.** 15 lb 15 oz
7. 18 lb 2 oz **8.** 7 tons 100 lb **9.** 14 tons 1400 lb **10.** 16 tons 100 lb **11.** 2 tons 1800 lb
12. 5 tons 1500 lb **13.** 52 oz **14.** $21\frac{1}{2}$ lb **15.** 9 oz **16.** $12\frac{7}{8}$ lb **17.** 13 oz
18. 820 lb

Objective 8.2C

1. 750 lb **2.** $15\frac{3}{4}$ ft **3.** 30 lb **4.** $1\frac{13}{16}$ ft **5.** 48 lb **6.** 27 lb **7.** 2 lb 8 oz
8. $7.15 **9.** $7.35 **10.** $30.24

Objective 8.3A

1. 3 c **2.** 16 fl oz **3.** 6 pt **4.** $3\frac{1}{2}$ pt **5.** 5 c **6.** 5 qt **7.** 5 gal

8. 3 gal **9.** 24 qt **10.** $4\frac{1}{2}$ qt **11.** 13 pt **12.** 20 qt **13.** 16 c **14.** 38 c

15. 15 c **16.** 72 fl oz **17.** 10 pt **18.** 13 c **19.** 12 qt **20.** 5 qt **21.** $2\frac{1}{2}$ pt

22. 40 qt **23.** 72 pt **24.** 48 fl oz **25.** 3 pt **26.** 8 gal **27.** $2\frac{3}{4}$ qt

Objective 8.3B

1. 3 qt 1 pt **2.** 5 qt 1 pt **3.** 5 qt **4.** 15 pt **5.** $13\frac{1}{2}$ gal **6.** 5 gal 3 qt **7.** 2 gal 2 qt
8. 3 c 5 fl oz **9.** 8 gal 2 qt **10.** 6 c 1 fl oz **11.** 1 gal 3 qt **12.** 2 gal 3 qt **13.** 14 qt **14.** 26 gal
15. 2 qt 1 pt **16.** 2 c 3 fl oz **17.** 8 c 2 fl oz **18.** 5 gal 1 qt

Objective 8.3C

1. 176 servings **2.** 22 qt **3.** 7 gal **4.** $3\frac{3}{4}$ c **5.** 6 gal **6.** $5\frac{1}{4}$ gal **7.** 21 pt

8. $12\frac{1}{2}$ lb **9.** Brand A **10.** $36.50

Objective 8.4A

1. 13 weeks **2.** 375 min **3.** $2\frac{1}{2}$ days **4.** $4\frac{1}{4}$ h **5.** 37 min **6.** 144 h **7.** 7 weeks

8. 315 days **9.** 17 h **10.** 64,800 s **11.** $3\frac{3}{4}$ days **12.** 7920 min **13.** 672 h **14.** 960 s

Objective 8.5A

1. 35,101 ft-lb **2.** 2,334,000 ft-lb **3.** 427,900 ft-lb **4.** 23,340,000 ft-lb **5.** 20,000 ft-lb **6.** 60,000 ft-lb
7. 48,000 ft-lb **8.** 192,000 ft-lb **9.** 600,000 ft-lb **10.** 8400 ft-lb **11.** 31,120,000 ft-lb
12. 58,350,000 ft-lb **13.** 11,670,000 ft-lb **14.** 960 ft-lb

Objective 8.5B

1. 12 hp **2.** 9 hp **3.** 5500 ft-lb/s **4.** 8250 ft-lb/s **5.** 2400 ft-lb/s **6.** 1800 ft-lb/s **7.** 12,000 ft-lb/s
8. 2000 ft-lb/s **9.** 1200 ft-lb/s **10.** 24 hp **11.** 10 hp **12.** 25 hp **13.** 32 hp **14.** 16 hp

CHAPTER 9

Objective 9.1A

1. 8.4 cm	**2.** 5.73 cm	**3.** 84,200 m	**4.** 1.96 m	**5.** 0.728 m	**6.** 642 cm	**7.** 830 m
8. 9.7 cm	**9.** 5.716 km	**10.** 23,128 m	**11.** 10,800 m	**12.** 0.825 m	**13.** 963 cm	**14.** 1260 mm
15. 24.3 cm	**16.** 17.66 cm	**17.** 5.713 km	**18.** 4218 m	**19.** 963 cm	**20.** 4.69 cm	**21.** 1960 mm
22. 7.539 km	**23.** 4218 m	**24.** 935 cm	**25.** 844 mm	**26.** 97,051 m	**27.** 179 mm	

Objective 9.1B

1. 33.6 m	**2.** 10.6 cm	**3.** 1.89 m	**4.** 9.4 m	**5.** 6.7 km	**6.** 49.4 m	**7.** 24.20 m
8. 12.7 m	**9.** $87.45	**10.** 3.25 km				

Objective 9.2A

1. 6.309 kg	**2.** 0.254 g	**3.** 0.058 g	**4.** 154 g	**5.** 560 mg	**6.** 2.754 kg	**7.** 3.248 g
8. 345 mg	**9.** 3910 g	**10.** 1.639 g	**11.** 22.8 mg	**12.** 980 mg	**13.** 975,000 mg	**14.** 0.086 g
15. 5400 g	**16.** 720 g	**17.** 0.854 kg	**18.** 0.634 kg	**19.** 0.038 g	**20.** 0.171 g	**21.** 7900 g
22. 123 g	**23.** 150 mg	**24.** 1,347,000 mg	**25.** 1856 g	**26.** 11.78 g	**27.** 317.084 g	

Objective 9.2B

1. 66.4 kg	**2.** 25.2 kg	**3.** 2.740 kg	**4.** 270 kg	**5.** 8 VCRs	**6.** $12.59	**7.** $450
8. $160	**9.** 120 kg	**10.** $42.25				

Objective 9.3A

1. 0.0058 L	**2.** 0.16 cm^3	**3.** 0.065 ml	**4.** 0.067 L	**5.** 1.038 L	**6.** 536 cm^3	**7.** 1650 cm^3
8. 2138 cm^3	**9.** 3325 cm^3	**10.** 4050 cm^3	**11.** 5738 cm^3	**12.** 9269 cm^3	**13.** 11,028 cm^3	**14.** 3310 L
15. 75 L	**16.** 2.347 kl	**17.** 2.7 L	**18.** 0.0032 L	**19.** 0.00684 kl	**20.** 2.076 L	**21.** 83 cm^3
22. 937 cm^3	**23.** 2679 cm^3	**24.** 4038 cm^3	**25.** 0.071 L	**26.** 1.036 L	**27.** 7.129 kl	

Objective 9.3B

1. 560.52 L	**2.** $0.385	**3.** 21.6 L	**4.** 12 L	**5.** 75 L	**6.** 1500 people	**7.** 9.3 L
8. 30 L	**9.** 16 containers	**10.** $122.40				

Objective 9.4A

1. 9800 Calories	**2.** 2800 Calories	**3.** 2730 Calories	**4.** 1555 Calories	**5.** $75.60
6. 2.79 kW h	**7.** 1000 wh	**8.** 4.55 kW h	**9.** $11.2896	**10.** 20%

Objective 9.5A

1. 200.2 m	**2.** 85 kg	**3.** 22.74 L	**4.** 58.87 L	**5.** 707 ml	**6.** 5.59 m	**7.** 96.6 km/h
8. 94.99 km/h	**9.** $6.38/kg	**10.** $3.28/kg	**11.** $1.27/L	**12.** $3.18/L	**13.** 1.21 lb	**14.** $0.54/L
15. 3542 km	**16.** 4950.75 km					

Objective 9.5B

1. 984 ft	**2.** 167.2 lb	**3.** 2.12 gal	**4.** 67.67 in.	**5.** 8200 ft	**6.** 17.64 oz	**7.** 16.89 gal
8. 1.57 in.	**9.** 1.92 pt	**10.** 47.20 mph	**11.** $1.23/gal	**12.** $1.95/lb	**13.** $1.53/gal	**14.** $6.04 gal
15. 7.29 hours	**16.** 0.84 lb					

CHAPTER 10

Objective 10.1A

1. +265   **2.** −5°   **3.** $-5\frac{3}{4}$ **4.** +5480

5.

```
←+--●--+--+--+--+--+--+--●--+--+→
 -5 -4 -3 -2 -1  0  1  2  3  4  5
```

6.

```
←+--+--+--+--+--+--●--●--+--+--+→
 -5 -4 -3 -2 -1  0  1  2  3  4  5
```

7.

```
←+--+--+--●--+--+--●--+--+--+--+→
 -5 -4 -3 -2 -1  0  1  2  3  4  5
```

8.

```
←+--+--●--+--●--+--+--+--+--+--+→
 -5 -4 -3 -2 -1  0  1  2  3  4  5
```

9. <   **10.** <   **11.** >   **12.** >   **13.** >   **14.** <   **15.** −15, −8, 2, 6   **16.** −5, 0, 7, 9   **17.** −9, 0, 3, 12

Objective 10.1B

1. −9   **2.** −3   **3.** 15   **4.** −65   **5.** 10   **6.** −3   **7.** 0.6   **8.** $2\frac{6}{7}$ **9.** −19   **10.** 28.1   **11.** $-\frac{5}{8}$ **12.** −9.7

13. <   **14.** <   **15.** >   **16.** <   **17.** =   **18.** >   **19.** −3, −1, 4, 6   **20.** −9, 3, 7, 10   **21.** −10, −6, 2, 5

Objective 10.2A

1. 8   **2.** −2   **3.** −6   **4.** −27   **5.** −41   **6.** 88   **7.** 3
8. −9   **9.** −8   **10.** −52   **11.** 0   **12.** 14   **13.** −14   **14.** −11
15. −13   **16.** 169   **17.** 59   **18.** −530   **19.** 10   **20.** 17   **21.** 20
22. −12   **23.** −19   **24.** −10

Objective 10.2B

1. 4   **2.** −11   **3.** −21   **4.** 79   **5.** −16   **6.** −203   **7.** −12
8. 15   **9.** 19   **10.** −74   **11.** 14   **12.** 45   **13.** 2   **14.** 1
15. 28   **16.** 34   **17.** −53   **18.** −19   **19.** −5   **20.** −4   **21.** −20
22. 4   **23.** 24   **24.** 19

Objective 10.2C

1. 0°C   **2.** −11°C   **3.** 259 points   **4.** 131 points   **5.** 3°F   **6.** 28°F   **7.** 42°F
8. 27°F   **9.** 9261 meters   **10.** 5670 meters

Objective 10.3A

1. −32   **2.** −56   **3.** 36   **4.** 99   **5.** 0   **6.** 493   **7.** −168
8. 504   **9.** −324   **10.** −384   **11.** −640   **12.** 0   **13.** −78   **14.** 52
15. 120   **16.** −115   **17.** −72   **18.** −126   **19.** 64   **20.** 90   **21.** −80

Objective 10.3B

1. −3   **2.** −9   **3.** 7   **4.** −4.63   **5.** −5   **6.** 13.33   **7.** 12
8. undefined   **9.** 5.31   **10.** −7.23   **11.** 25.68   **12.** 17.83   **13.** −47   **14.** 0
15. 29   **16.** −12   **17.** −84   **18.** 70   **19.** −14   **20.** 4   **21.** −70

Objective 10.3C

1. −3   **2.** −7°C   **3.** −14°C   **4.** −7   **5.** −0.82   **6.** −0.54   **7.** 94   **8.** 96

Objective 10.4A

1. $-1\frac{1}{12}$ **2.** $\frac{4}{9}$ **3.** $\frac{22}{35}$ **4.** $-\frac{35}{36}$ **5.** $-1\frac{17}{24}$ **6.** $-6\frac{65}{72}$ **7.** 3.6

8. -17.32 **9.** -11.798 **10.** -17.9 **11.** 5.88   **12.** 10.824   **13.** $-1\frac{11}{24}$ **14.** $\frac{8}{15}$

15. $\frac{5}{44}$ **16.** $7\frac{3}{5}$ **17.** -30.27 **18.** -9.056 **19.** 18.94   **20.** -7.372 **21.** 8.95

Objective 10.4B

1. $-\frac{1}{4}$ **2.** $\frac{7}{27}$ **3.** $-\frac{5}{24}$ **4.** 2   **5.** -12 **6.** $-4\frac{4}{9}$ **7.** 16.74

8. -95.94 **9.** -132.6 **10.** $-\frac{8}{9}$ **11.** $-1\frac{1}{4}$ **12.** $\frac{2}{3}$ **13.** $-\frac{2}{5}$ **14.** $\frac{5}{9}$ **15.** $-1\frac{3}{4}$

Objective 10.4C

1. 39.99°F   **2.** 22.23°F   **3.** 161.4°F   **4.** \$8.18   **5.** \$158.11   **6.** 26.12°F   **7.** \$53.57
8. \$77.32

Objective 10.5A

1. 4.2×10^{5} **2.** 7.9×10^{-6} **3.** 3.62×10^{9} **4.** 8.2×10^{10} **5.** 8.1×10^{-8} **6.** 1.54×10^{-7} **7.** 6.6×10^{-9}
8. 7.385×10^{8} **9.** 0.0000463   **10.** 69,500,000   **11.** 25,760,000,000   **12.** 0.0000000129   **13.** 9,110,000
14. 573,000,000   **15.** 0.000378   **16.** 0.000000714

Objective 10.5B

1. 10   **2.** 1   **3.** -38 **4.** -39 **5.** -1 **6.** 5   **7.** 20
8. -20 **9.** -13 **10.** 147   **11.** 5.8   **12.** -16 **13.** -18.63 **14.** -18.86
15. -2.94 **16.** $1\frac{1}{2}$

CHAPTER 11

Objective 11.1A

1. 2   **2.** 7   **3.** -10 **4.** -10 **5.** -11 **6.** 11   **7.** -22
8. 7   **9.** 1   **10.** -40 **11.** -9 **12.** 4   **13.** 16   **14.** 22
15. -3 **16.** -3 **17.** 2   **18.** 16   **19.** 2   **20.** -14 **21.** $1\frac{1}{2}$
22. 15   **23.** 9   **24.** -21 **25.** 29   **26.** 11   **27.** 14

Objective 11.1B

1. $14a$ **2.** $11x$ **3.** $-8y$ **4.** $-7mn$ **5.** $13x^{2}$ **6.** $10x-3$ **7.** $4t$

8. y **9.** $-5uv$ **10.** $6y^{2}-xy$ **11.** $6x^{2}-3$ **12.** $12w-6u$ **13.** $-14ab$ **14.** $5x^{2}-5y^{2}$

15. $-2xy-6y$ **16.** $-6ab-4a$ **17.** $5x^{2}-y$ **18.** $6y$ **19.** $15y^{2}-7y$ **20.** $-4x+5y$ **21.** $-4w+5v$

22. $3m+14n$ **23.** $-3z-4y$ **24.** $-6ab+4ac$ **25.** $22x^{2}-2x$ **26.** $3a^{2}-8ab$ **27.** $-11x^{2}+7x$

Answers to Drill-and-Practice Pages

Objective 11.1C

1. $3x + 6$	**2.** $5m + 20$	**3.** $7y - 14$	**4.** $-3a - 9$	**5.** $-4a - 20$	**6.** $9x - 9y$	**7.** $-2x + 2$
8. $15x - 5$	**9.** $12x + 32$	**10.** $6m - 15$	**11.** $-2w + 10$	**12.** $-4v + 36$	**13.** $4a - 4b$	**14.** $8m - 24$
15. $14a - 7$	**16.** $5x - 12$	**17.** $4x + 8$	**18.** $5x + 7$	**19.** 6	**20.** $9m + 15$	**21.** $-x + 35$
22. $5y + 13$	**23.** $a - 5$	**24.** $16x + 3$	**25.** $16x - 4$	**26.** $-5y - 6$	**27.** $x - 6$	

Objective 11.2A

1. Yes	**2.** No	**3.** Yes	**4.** No	**5.** Yes	**6.** Yes	**7.** Yes
8. Yes	**9.** Yes	**10.** No	**11.** No	**12.** Yes	**13.** Yes	**14.** No
15. Yes	**16.** Yes	**17.** No	**18.** Yes	**19.** Yes	**20.** No	

Objective 11.2B

1. $x = 6$	**2.** $n = 3$	**3.** $x = -4$	**4.** $w = -7$	**5.** $x = -4$	**6.** $x = 0$	**7.** $t = 2$
8. $v = 4$	**9.** $x = 3$	**10.** $x = 1$	**11.** $y = -5$	**12.** $x = 17$	**13.** $y = 10$	**14.** $x = -11$
15. $t = -5$	**16.** $x = -9$	**17.** $t = -7$	**18.** $w = -11$	**19.** $z = 2$	**20.** $x = -11$	**21.** $x = -\frac{1}{2}$
22. $x = \frac{2}{7}$	**23.** $y = -\frac{2}{3}$	**24.** $y = -\frac{3}{4}$	**25.** $x = 11$	**26.** $x = 6.4$	**27.** $x = -7$	

Objective 11.2C

1. $x = 4$	**2.** $x = 5$	**3.** $x = -2$	**4.** $t = -8$	**5.** $y = 6$	**6.** $y = -7$	**7.** $y = 4$
8. $y = -7$	**9.** $x = 20$	**10.** $x = 27$	**11.** $n = -18$	**12.** $x = -30$	**13.** $x = -10$	**14.** $m = -24$
15. $x = 12$	**16.** $y = 6$	**17.** $x = 14$	**18.** $v = -6$	**19.** $x = -20$	**20.** $w = -50$	**21.** $z = 12$
22. $x = 24$	**23.** $x = -64$	**24.** $y = 36$	**25.** $t = -16$	**26.** $x = -42$	**27.** $a = 28$	

Objective 11.2D

1. $31,250	**2.** $4800	**3.** $180	**4.** $45	**5.** 25%	**6.** 20%	**7.** $6000	**8.** $800

Objective 11.3A

1. $x = 3$	**2.** $x = 7$	**3.** $x = -2$	**4.** $x = 6$	**5.** $x = -3$	**6.** $x = 1$	**7.** $x = 3$
8. $x = 7$	**9.** $x = 2$	**10.** $x = -6$	**11.** $x = 7$	**12.** $x = -1$	**13.** $x = -5$	**14.** $x = 7$
15. $x = -1$	**16.** $x = -7$	**17.** $x = 3$	**18.** $x = -1$	**19.** $x = -3$	**20.** $x = 20$	**21.** $x = 7$
22. $x = 5$	**23.** $x = 2$	**24.** $x = 3$	**25.** $x = -1$	**26.** $x = 3$	**27.** $x = -2$	

Objective 11.3B

1. $203°F$	**2.** $-7.6°F$	**3.** 600 tables	**4.** 4000 blenders	**5.** $3520	**6.** $80,000

7. $2\frac{1}{4}$ seconds   **8.** $22\frac{3}{4}$ seconds

Objective 11.4A

1. $x = -5$	**2.** $x = -3$	**3.** $x = -8$	**4.** $x = -3$	**5.** $x = 2$	**6.** $x = -1$	**7.** $x = 6$
8. $x = 2$	**9.** $x = 1$	**10.** $x = 3$	**11.** $x = -6$	**12.** $x = 6$	**13.** $x = 3$	**14.** $x = -9$
15. $x = -1$	**16.** $x = 3$	**17.** $x = 6$	**18.** $x = 10$	**19.** $x = 0$	**20.** $x = 2$	**21.** $x = -2$
22. $x = 12$	**23.** $x = 2$	**24.** $x = -2$				

Objective 11.4B

1. $x = -5$ **2.** $x = 1$ **3.** $x = -1\frac{1}{2}$ **4.** $x = -6$ **5.** $x = 6$ **6.** $x = -21$ **7.** $x = -13$

8. $x = 2$ **9.** $x = 3$ **10.** $x = 1$ **11.** $x = 24$ **12.** $x = 10$ **13.** $x = 2$ **14.** $x = 6$

15. $x = 7$ **16.** $x = 3$ **17.** $x = -1$ **18.** $x = 12$ **19.** $x = 1$ **20.** $x = 1$ **21.** $x = 8$

22. $x = 8$ **23.** $x = -1$ **24.** $x = 0$

Objective 11.5A

1. $x + 8$ **2.** $c - 3$ **3.** $5x$ **4.** $\dfrac{y}{c}$ **5.** $2(m + n)$ **6.** $m - n$ **7.** $x + x^3$

8. $v - 2v^2$ **9.** $x + \dfrac{1}{2}y$ **10.** $a\left(\dfrac{a}{3}\right)$ **11.** $x - x^2$ **12.** $x(x + 3)$ **13.** $\dfrac{x-1}{x}$ **14.** $x + \dfrac{x}{5}$

15. $\dfrac{y}{y+1}$ **16.** $\dfrac{y+1}{y}$ **17.** $c + 2c$ **18.** $\dfrac{1}{6}m - m$ **19.** $\dfrac{b}{3+b}$ **20.** $xy + 4$ **21.** $x - 3x$

Objective 11.5B

1. $t + 8$ **2.** $x - 6$ **3.** $y - 6$ **4.** $-3z$ **5.** $\dfrac{1}{2}c + c$ **6.** $r + r^2$ **7.** $m(m + 2)$

8. $a - 2a$ **9.** $x + \dfrac{x}{3}$ **10.** $m\left(\dfrac{1}{3}m\right)$ **11.** $\dfrac{h+4}{h}$ **12.** $x + 7x^2$ **13.** $x(x+1)$ **14.** $\dfrac{1}{5}x - 1$

15. x^3 **16.** $m + 11$ **17.** $n - 2$ **18.** $3n$ **19.** $\dfrac{n}{12}$ **20.** $\dfrac{2}{3}n$ **21.** $2 + n$

Objective 11.6A

1. $4x = 24; x = 6$ **2.** $\dfrac{x}{6} = 5; x = 30$ **3.** $x + 9 = 1; x = -8$ **4.** $\dfrac{x}{12} = 3; x = 36$

5. $5x = 24; x = 4\dfrac{4}{5}$ **6.** $\dfrac{2}{3}x = 18; x = 9$ **7.** $x + 11 = 4; x = -7$ **8.** $2x + 5 = 13; x = 4$

9. $\dfrac{1}{4}x + 5 = 8; x = 12$ **10.** $4x - 5 = 11; x = 4$ **11.** $\dfrac{x}{3} + 4 = 2; x = -6$ **12.** $\dfrac{x}{8} + 10 = 2; x = -64$

13. $\dfrac{x}{7} = 11; x = 77$ **14.** $4 + 2x = 40; x = 19$ **15.** $6 + \dfrac{x}{4} = -3; x = -36$ **16.** $1 - \dfrac{x}{5} = 2; x = -5$

Objective 11.6B

1. $T + \$158 = \$2640; T = \$2482$ **2.** $P + \$20 = \$99; P = \$79$ **3.** $P + 0.16P = \$130{,}500; P = \$112{,}500$

4. $0.15P = \$60; P = \$400$ **5.** $0.10P = 40{,}000, P = 400{,}000$ **6.** $C + 0.33C = \$119.40; C = \$89.77$

7. $0.01S = \$1000; S = \$100{,}000$ **8.** $30P = \$1950; P = \$65$ **9.** $65A = 1040; A = 16$ squares

10. $\dfrac{1}{10}S = \$150; S = \$1500$